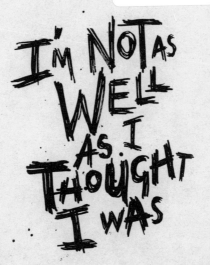

I'M NOT AS
WELL
AS I
THOUGHT
I WAS

RUBY WAX

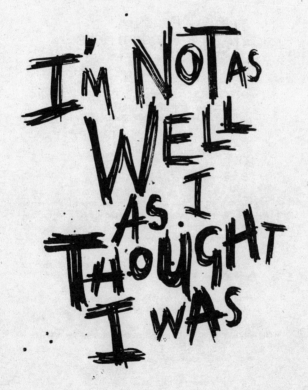

I'M NOT AS WELL AS I THOUGHT I WAS

LIFE

PENGUIN LIFE

UK | USA | Canada | Ireland | Australia
India | New Zealand | South Africa

Penguin Life is part of the Penguin Random House group of companies
whose addresses can be found at global.penguinrandomhouse.com.

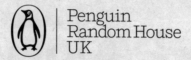

First published 2023
This edition published 2024
001

Typeset by Jouve (UK), Milton Keynes
Printed and bound in Great Britain by Clays Ltd, Elcograf S.p.A.

The authorized representative in the EEA is Penguin Random House Ireland,
Morrison Chambers, 32 Nassau Street, Dublin D02 YH68

A CIP catalogue record for this book is available from the British Library

ISBN: 978–0–241–55491–3

www.greenpenguin.co.uk

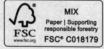

MIX
Paper | Supporting
responsible forestry
FSC® C018179

Penguin Random House is committed to a
sustainable future for our business, our readers
and our planet. This book is made from Forest
Stewardship Council® certified paper.

To my brilliant editor, Alison Summers, without whom this book would be an incomprehensible rant.

To my wonderful therapist, Priscilla Short.

To my equally wonderful psychiatrist, James Arkell.

To my family, who stand by me no matter how nuts I go.

Contents

1

The Clinic

I've spent a lifetime creating a 'front' to give the illusion that all is well. It wasn't, and it isn't.

– RW

Clinic

11 May 2022

BANG! BANG! BANG! BANG! BANG! BANG! This was the only sound I could hear each day while getting a treatment called Repetitive, Transcranial, Magnetic Stimulation. Some young guy wearing an apron like he's a butcher, not a doctor, put something like a bathing cap over my head and strapped it under my chin. Then something that looked like a 50s hairdryer was lowered over my head.

But it's not a hairdryer, it's way more than a hairdryer. It's a complex piece of machinery that stimulates the brain and causes 'neuroplasticity'. Picture 82 billion strands of spaghetti (they're neurons, in case someone out there is believing our heads are full of pasta) changing partners, making new connections (trillions of them) with every zap of the hammer. Like speed-dating but for neurons.

It feels like Woody Woodpecker and his cartoon pals are

gang-banging my head. And it Bangs! Bangs! Bangs! fast and furious. You get eighteen pulses in one second and that happens fifty-five times in a session. I can't do the maths, but it's a lot of zaps. I am so desperate, I don't mind the bangs even though they're pretty violent. If you've had Botox, this is nothing.

He knows it's working when my face contorts. It suddenly twitches into a grotesque grimace and he tells me that's a sign it's doing its job. I always like to compete even with myself, so I tell him to up the intensity, which he does, and my face turns into a tight convulsive pucker – a gurn. I figure if the hammering is set higher, I won't have to do twenty. I'm wrong. You do have to do all twenty sessions.

Remember that scene when Dr Frankenstein is using the power of an electrical storm outside as voltage to wake up his monster and get him walking with the ridiculous 'goose steps and sleepwalker arms'? Of course you do. After the first treatment, I walk like that along madhouse hallways with the blue, frayed, badly stained industrial carpets. When was this place last decorated? Good question. There's a painting of Florence Nightingale on the wall, so my guess is she must have personally helped them with the decor and colour schemes.

If you would have told me that something like rTMS existed, I'd think you had watched too much sci-fi. rTMS, unlike ECT (electroconvulsive therapy), is the 'last saloon' treatment for those who don't respond to any medication. With ECT they knock you out, put a bit between your teeth so you don't bite off your tongue, and let the voltage rip. Electric currents bring on a small seizure which, fingers crossed, changes the brain chemistry. In other words, you're fried, and even worse, there's a good chance that there might be a tiny bit of memory loss. Not good for any human who wants to remember their name or if they're from Planet Earth. rTMS uses magnets which have no serious side-effects but it's still a jump-start for the neurons to communicate better.

I don't answer my phone because I wouldn't know who I am, let alone who they are. Nothing is working except my eyes, which dart around the room. I notice they designed it to make sure there's nothing you could hang yourself from. There are no faucets in the sink, so water squirts from the wall. How do you hang yourself from a faucet? There are plastic hangers which can't even hang on a rail, so most of them are on the floor. I could think of a few ways if you wanted to end your life, as in butt your head into the television screen. But I'm not thinking about killing myself. I just wish my life would stop. It hurts so much.

There's a constant stream of nurses coming in to see me. Some take blood, some hand me little cups filled with multi-coloured pills, some come to check I'm still alive, some to bring me food which tastes like Styrofoam. The only thing identifiable is corn, otherwise it's all brown lumps. It's brought to me three times a day, wrapped in cellophane. The cellophane is the most delicious part.

Did I mention that the elevator doesn't work? It's been stuck between the second and third floor for about forty-five minutes today. The person who I would say is the most unstable of us all is in it. We can hear the screams throughout the building, but the nurses assure us it's just someone stuck in an elevator. It's not our imagination, which would be far worse.

In case you haven't realized by now, I'm writing this from a mental institution. My room has all the charm of the hotel room/prison I was isolated in at Heathrow Airport after entering the UK from South Africa during Covid times. There, at the Holiday Inn Exchange, I paid a mere £1,200 for the privilege of being incarcerated for twelve days in a box. The view was a roundabout at Terminal 4. I'd wait with excitement each day for a truck to loop around; sometimes it went around twice. The food was imaginative – think of eating chicken topped with fingernail clippings.

I haven't taken a shower because of the missing shower head that they removed in case I try to hang myself if the faucet doesn't work on the sink. Water just squirts out from the ceiling in every direction but not on me, so I've stopped taking showers.

At night the only thing that gives me any joy, as the sleeping pills work their magic, is cramming chocolate digestive biscuits into my mouth while watching all the seasons of *Friends* back to back. I like the colours in the apartment where Rachel and Monica are living. One of their walls is purple. That's my favourite colour. I can't really understand the plots so I must be far gone. I'm on the Chocolate Digestive Biscuit Diet. I woke up this morning with chocolate smeared all over my face.

The nurses are from agencies, so they don't really specialize in mental illness – or anything else as far as I can tell. Today someone dressed as half nurse, half cleaning woman came into my room and told me that if I gave myself depression, I should be able to get myself out of it. It was her expert opinion that I should put on my trousers, get out of bed and back out to where I came from. So I went screaming down the hallway to the nurses' station, 'What are we in, some born-again Christian cult?' Anyway, she came in later to apologize: 'Sorry, I just heard you're a mental health advocate.' (She says the word 'advocate' as if it's unfamiliar territory. Clearly, it's the first time she's used it; she probably thinks it means avocado.) She continues, 'Please tell me how to deal with somebody with mental illness. What are the steps?' You'd think getting a professional mental health worker might be included in the price of a room.

Checking in here wasn't exactly on my agenda. Writing about it, even less so, yet here we are. I come from a long line of ancestors with various flavours of mental illness, so genetically it seems to be a no-brainer that I'd be the next in line. But, after twelve years of no depression, I have to admit it took me by surprise. I had stayed clean. I mean, there were little spurts of darkness prior to this but I always managed to put out the fires by recognizing the signs early and doing something to ward it off. This time I hadn't noticed the speed picking up or that toxic fog rolling into my brain or the sense of sinking in quicksand.

The Big Dip snuck up on me and when it did, it struck hard. Depression is the black hole of diseases, where you sit helpless as your mind hammers you with accusations. Your thoughts attack like little demons biting chunks out of your brain. It's hard to stay alive and listen. But I can write, because by some miracle my hands can type without the use of my mind. It's as if they have a life of their own. *I type, therefore I am.*

My too short orange curtains are permanently closed because the sunlight burns my eyes as if I am a vampire. My mind is a cacophony of shrieks from Hell. I can't even hear my own thoughts because it's so loud in there.

If I peek out, I see a main street with normal life going on. Everyone outside seems to know where they're going, whether it's appointments, jobs, or lunches with friends. It seems unimaginable that I once knew where I was going too.

They're so lucky: they still believe they live in some kind of reality, whereas I'm not too sure there is one. I can't tell if something is taking a few minutes or hours, my mind is white noise.

12 May 2022

Today I have to do a corporate gig where I talk to a business over Zoom. This gig was booked two months earlier and I didn't want to cancel, even though Ed tells me it's insane to do a talk to 700 people online when I'm insane. Do I listen to him? Never. Before it starts, I try to put makeup on but my hand is shaking too much. When I check, I see there is mascara on my lower lip.

I try to adjust the camera so no one can tell I'm in a mental clinic, but a large hospital bed might be a giveaway. Somebody online introduces me, and for a second I don't know who I am. Then I talk for an hour about stigma and why we should break it, while leaving out the elephant in the room. That's me, who has depression, and isn't mentioning it.

At one point during Q and A someone asks, 'How do you know when someone has depression?' I should have shoved my face in the camera and said, 'It looks like this,' but I didn't. Just as I think I might get away with it, the door flies open and a nurse enters holding my drugs on her tray and announces it's time for my medication. I get up and literally shove her out the door. After the experience was over, and I was covered in sweat and panting, I decided maybe Ed was right about not doing any more online talks while I'm here.

Ed visits. Ed has become my own personal sherpa. Usually as soon as he makes a delivery, I hand him a new list and he doesn't complain. This time I've asked him to bring me pyjamas, raisins, bran flakes and writing paper. He's always smiling and perky. Today this pisses me off. Why is he so happy? What chemicals has he got in his veins that I don't have? Why do I have to be medicated and drugged to get where he is naturally?

I've been told there is a library here, and that I'm allowed to bring books to my room. But I can't read anything. When I look at words, the letters aren't in the right order. All I can do is watch Anthony Bourdain on the television over and over. When I look under his smiling, eating exterior, I get the sense Bourdain doesn't feel at home anywhere either, and that's why he keeps moving to one location after another. I'm guessing he's not travelling the world for ambition's sake but just to be on the move.

Moving is my oxygen, too. Like a great white shark, I never stop gliding, always hunting. I'm always looking for something. I don't know what it is or even where it is. It doesn't matter what I've accomplished, I need to jump over the next hurdle, and the next. I know I've had success, yes, thank you, take a bow. But I never think about those things. I certainly don't feel them.

I reinvented myself, and I've prided myself on reinvention ever since. People go, 'Wow, that's so impressive.' Reinvention is such a positive word. But for me, each reinvention was just another form of escape. My biggest fear was grinding to a halt, unable to go anywhere: a paralysed lump in the custody of my parents. Reinvention was a survival tactic, grabbing for a life jacket that keeps slipping out of reach. Now I look back at all my reinventions and think, 'What the fuck was I thinking?'

The last film made about Bourdain is a biography called *Roadrunner*. It leads up to his death. When they interviewed all his friends, they seemed shocked. They say he was so full of life, and he had the greatest job on earth: going around the world, meeting people and eating. That does seem like a dream job, but as the thousands of seasons go on, I can see a weariness come into his eyes and it's the look I have in my eyes.

Towards the end of the film, all joy is gone. Travelling the world, meeting new people, even eating doesn't do it for him. They finally find him hanging by his belt. I think I saw it coming. He was running from one experience to the next, but nothing was registering. Nothing stuck.

Before I came to the clinic, I'd been on medication for several decades. The psychiatrist who'd prescribed the medication said it was time to rethink the recipe because it seemed not to be working. Duh! Then he said he was prepared to change my medication but that he also wanted me to talk to a therapist who specializes in trauma.

I always assumed trauma was an 'Oprah' word. I thought only people who fought in Iraq or Afghanistan had trauma, while I had inherited depression from my seriously demented family tree. I thought it was inevitable. I come from a long line of insane ancestors, probably beginning millions of years ago with a crazy single cell. And that's just on my mother's side. Many of the relatives on my father's side enjoyed a buffet of schizophrenia, bi-polar, and personality disorders. They didn't even have to wait for a war to kill them, they killed themselves first.

But the psychiatrist kept insisting I had trauma. He said while I was in the clinic, he wanted me to see a therapist who did EMDR. When I asked what that was, he said, 'eye movement desensitization and reprocessing'. This was pure gobbledegook to me; just more letters jumping around.

He described it as a form of therapy where you follow a pendulum moving right to left and back again. Okay, I thought, now he's really taking the piss. But he insisted it worked for trauma. (Maybe it does if you have it, which I don't.) Anyway, I finally gave in. I said I would try this EMDR but only if he promised to change the meds.

13 May 2022

Shrink session

The shrink is a young-looking middle-aged woman with a kind, almost cute face, and sharp eyes behind brown-framed glasses. Her hair could be light blonde or white depending on the light. She sits at a desk with nothing on it but her notebook. Over her head there's an app that makes an online ball for the EMDR process that goes back and forth across the screen. I hope I don't go blind.

S: I want you to follow the ball on the screen and –

R: Is that ball going to keep going back and forth because I may get seasick.

S: Tell me where you picture yourself as a child growing up?

R: Okay, as a child where else would I be? I'm at my house in Evanston, Illinois. Land of Lincoln as seen on a penny. I'm in my bedroom, which is spooky. Everyone thought it was, not just me.

S: Are you in bed?

R: No, I'm sitting on the floor. I can't lie on the bed because my mother has made it up. She has the bedspread perfectly placed on top, all its creases are straightened, and the sheets pulled tight. I'm not allowed to lie on it until after she unmakes it at night.

S: What else do you see?

R: There is a chest of drawers. I'm forbidden to open the drawers in case everything in there gets rumpled. At night, she pulls all my clothes out of the drawers and then she refolds them back in.

S: How old are you in this image?

R: Four, five. Why are you asking me that? I never tell anyone my age.

S: Look around. What else do you see in your bedroom?

R: Everything's creepy, I told you. There's a bookshelf with a musical merry-go-round on it with little German fairytale figures.

S: Tell me what you're feeling as you revisit your old bedroom.

R: I'm feeling like this isn't going anywhere. It's not like I can go back and redecorate my room.

S: It's only through recognizing the feelings you had at the time that you can let go of pain from the past.

R: Yeah, blah blah shrink stuff. (I think it but I don't say it.)

S: No matter how much you try to repress it, your past affects how you are.

R: I don't have trauma, just a shit background.

S: Can you describe the rest of the house to me?

R: It's like a haunted house. I don't mean like the cute one in Disneyland, but a deadly one where you never get out alive.

S: *What about your mother? Where is she in the house?*

R: *She is walking around upstairs with wide, thundering strides. Sometimes the floor would shake. When I was little, I imagined a witch taking big strides like that, and I couldn't always tell whether she was my mother or a witch. The house was only quiet when she was in her bathroom. She sometimes stayed there for hours. For me that was a good day. I don't know what she was doing in her bathroom; making a brew maybe?*

S: *Where is your father in the house?*

R: *The living room. He listens to Wagner at full blast to drown out my mother's screams about what 'morons' we are.*

S: *Tell me about the house rules.*

R: *I was allowed to watch TV in our basement. The basement looked like a bierkeller/Nazi hangout.*

S: *What do you mean?*

R: *The walls were dark wood panelling; there were cuckoo clocks and stuffed dead animals on the walls. My parents also collected grotesque German corkscrews: warty wooden old men's heads with corkscrews for bodies. Only the Germans could think up that. I wasn't allowed to go into the attic. I would have been too scared anyway. I thought all the dead relatives left behind in Vienna were there cocooned in spiderwebs. And I couldn't sit on the porch. I don't remember why. I wasn't allowed in my parents' bedroom in case I touched anything. I once opened a drawer and found a finger. I'm joking, there was no finger.*

Actually, this is one of the few times I've spoken about my parents without trying to be funny. I usually tell stories about them in comedy speak. They've always given me my best material. I didn't even have to edit what they said, every line went straight from their lips to my page.

S: *Let's continue without the comedy. You mentioned a merry-go-round on the bookshelf in your bedroom. Go with that image, and notice what comes up.*

R: *When I was a teenager, and fighting with my mother, one of us would always end up throwing it across the room to smash it against the wall. Eventually it was just limbs hanging from metal stumps, or headless torsos in dirndls. But it never stopped going round and round with that plink plink kiddy music. I can still hear the sound it made.*

I hadn't thought about any of this stuff for a long time. Talking about it brought back the feeling that I had as a child: that I was a freak, with freak parents, living a freakish life.

When I turned off the Zoom I thought, 'What am I doing following a ball going across a screen?' It was like I was playing a tiny tennis game.

*

Ed comes to deliver the raisins he forgot to deliver last time. I want to tip him and then I remember I'm married to him, and I don't have to. I remind him he also forgot my extra socks, pyjamas and underwear, because now I know I'm staying longer. He starts to write it all down.

I've watched all the seasons of *Anthony Bourdain* and *Friends* so there's nothing else to do. The hallway is where the action is, so I've started to bravely walk across my room and open my door a crack. A young pregnant girl does her Zombie walk, up and down the passageway, clutching her half-eaten teddy bear. I take another step and watch someone having an argument with the air. Who do they imagine they're shouting at? A boyfriend? A policeman? A ghost?

14 May 2022

Shrink session

I'm glad I know nothing about the shrink. This is the way it should be. Otherwise, I'd spend every session doing what I always do: comparing myself, judging her and envying her sanity. But this way she's just another brain trying to help me figure out mine. Which doesn't mean I won't try and guess what her life's like, but so far, I haven't got many clues.

S: *When did you start turning your family experiences into comedy?*

R: *It was around thirty years ago. I was flying to Chicago to see my parents around six times a year. After I'd get back to Heathrow, I'd take a bus straight away to Alan Rickman's house in Shepherd's Bush.*

S: *The actor?*

R: *Yes. We became best friends when we were in the Royal Shakespeare Company together. We shared a house in Stratford-upon-Avon. We named it 'Shakespeare's Spa and Sauna' because some of the walls were covered in tin foil.*

We also shared a tortoise called Betty. I once tried to get Betty a part in Antony and Cleopatra. I stopped Peter Brook, the director, in the street and asked him if he'd let Betty audition for the role of the asp. Alan was with me. I mentioned she wouldn't have a problem playing it nude. Alan pretended not to know me, but we laughed about it afterwards.

S: You were telling me about stopping at his place, after arriving back at Heathrow.

R: That's right. After I got to Alan's house, I'd do a three-hour monologue about my parents and how insane they were. When I made Alan laugh, that was the equivalent of winning an Oscar. He was very selective about what he found funny, but my parents soon became his favourite comedy bit. I'd be drinking and smoking and monologuing like I was on stage in Vegas. Then I'd pass out on his sofa, and his partner Rima would cover me with a blanket. This was a tradition that went on for more than ten years.

S: You said you went six times a year. Why did you take so many trips to Chicago?

R: They bribed me. My father would tell me I was an heiress and when he died, I would inherit a fortune. That's why I never told them to fuck off, which I should have.

My dad would go, 'Boy, have you got a lot of money. What are you going to do with all that money?' Then he'd take me to the bank in downtown Evanston to the safety deposit room and make me stand about ten feet away and then crinkle some papers going, 'That's your will! Boy, are you going to be rich.' So I stuck around. (I didn't become an heiress as promised.)

With Alan watching as my audience, it's like I was exorcizing the effect my parents had on me. If I could make the experience I'd *just had in Evanston funny, I didn't have to feel the humiliation of it. Being funny is probably the only reason I wasn't committed a long time ago. Being funny means I can attract people to keep me feeling protected and safe.*

*

A few hours ago, I put my head around my door to see what was going on in the drug dispensary. Everyone in the queue is always swapping medication, either to get high or to put themselves to sleep. Recently, the nurses have gotten wise to this one, so now people have to swallow the pills in front of them and open their mouths wide to show they went down. But the staff are often so distracted, they wouldn't notice if you pulled a crocodile out of your mouth. The nurses are usually in a flap, getting everyone's meds wrong. Some inmates are now taking photos of the bottles to make sure it's what they've been prescribed. Smart move.

15 May 2022

Shrink session

Today the shrink has changed location at her house. She is sitting in a pinewood-panelled room, identical to our Germanic basement in Evanston except without the stuffed dead animals and cuckoo clocks on the walls. I ask her next time to change back to her regular room with the white walls to stop me having any flashbacks.

S: *I've been thinking about how you used humour to deal with your trauma. It was very effective in keeping you safe for many years.*

R: *But not any more. Look where I am.*

S: *Let's see if there's a way you can deal with trauma that doesn't involve laughing at it, but rather facing it. Because we can't fix things if we don't face them. It won't be easy, and it will take time. We will need to process the trauma in a way that's within your zone of tolerance.*

There is a bookshelf behind her. I try to squint to see what she reads but it's too far away.

S: *I'd like to hear more about where you lived. Without the comedy.*

R: *Why? It's the better version.*

S: *Just try and leave it out during our working together.*

R: *Okay, I'll try, but if it gets boring, let me know. I came from Evanston and we lived next to Lake Michigan. I thought Russia was on the other side and I used to collect berries and bury them in case we were ever attacked. Waking life was sad. I remember sitting with my dog in front of the big picture window looking out. Our house faced a park which would be filled with families on the weekends, bbq-ing burgers and hotdogs and everybody was laughing and the mom was mixing coleslaw and the kids were throwing balls and my dog and I really wanted to be part of that normal life. Actually, I don't know what my dog was thinking. Maybe the same as me. Or meeting that special dog. I guess what I'm saying is that as a child I was extremely lonely, and so was my dog.*

S: *Would you tell me some more about being a little girl growing up in the Evanston house?*

R: *Okay, if it will make you happy. The house was always dark. In my nightmares I run to the light switches one after the other* *because someone's coming for me in our house, and none of them work. I'm panicking, flicking all of them on and off and nothing happens, no light.*

S: *Who did you think was after you?*

R: *I don't think someone was after me, I know someone was after me. Always my dad. I had a fight with him once when I was fifteen years old. I told him to shut up, and he called me a brat, and took a swing. I made a bolt to the front door and ran. He chased me across the street to a girl's house, Linda Schwartz. I wasn't friends with her – she was very popular at school – but I took a chance she'd be home. Linda was having a party with the other popular girls but after banging on the door, she let me in. I burst into the living room with my dad chasing me and I huddled in a corner while he was trying to kick me. The girls surrounded me, forming a kind of human igloo to stop him, but he kept kicking me between their legs. After he finally went, all the girls went back to eating potato chips, silently, not looking at me. I was so embarrassed. They didn't ask me to join them. I apologized for making a scene and I left. I knew they would gossip about me. They'd say I was a weirdo, and they'd be right. I was so ashamed. I can still feel the humiliation loud and clear. From then on, I always felt like an outsider.*

S: *No child should have that happen.*

*

Even though I can't believe in the magic of the bouncing ball with EMDR, I suppose the shrink has helped me realize that I've created a funny personality to cover up the fact that most of the time I feel empty and rudderless. I spent a lifetime creating a 'front' to give the illusion that all was well. I built myself some pretty impenetrable armour. I look back at my life and think, 'What the fuck was that all about?'

I didn't set out to write a book about being in a mental clinic. It was going to be a kind of guide for people who wanted to find something deeper in their lives: find a purpose outside a job and a partner and living the 'same old, same old'.

Ambition served me well in the first half of my life, with hot and cold running success and attention. But at a certain age if you don't go deeper, you're at the mercy of watching yourself age with no rewards. I wanted to age with some benefits, otherwise what's the point? That's exactly what I wanted to find out by writing this book – The Point. So I started writing about going on journeys with the intention of finding meaning, purpose to life, peace, compassion, joy – whatever you want to call it.

I had booked various journeys to find all those things, or at least one or two of them. Later I found out it was ludicrous to be setting myself up as some kind of expert, a sort of sage who would know where to find meaning. I don't know what meaning even means. Obviously, it's different things to different people. Who am I to say what gives meaning? Look, if you're in the Ukraine and you dodge a missile and get out, that's meaning enough. Other people might just want to be cosy on a sofa with their family watching the telly. (See Gogglebox.) Other people would think this 'meaning' thing is bollocks.

These were some of my journeys:

SPIRIT ROCK: A month-long silent retreat at Spirit Rock – a killer. The Iron Man of mindfulness, but after all hard-core discipline, I thought I might find some meaning.

Not to be confused with the book about mindfulness through origami, 'Mind-foldness'.

HUMPBACKS: I thought, 'Throw yourself into the deep end, Ruby, and go swimming with the biggest whales you can find.' Who knows? It might give you a little more humility and a lot less ego. It could be a life-changer.

A REFUGEE CAMP: I said to myself, 'Stop being so self-ish and do something for someone else for a change.' That's a new one for me. I worked in a refugee camp in Greece to stoke up on compassion.

A CHRISTIAN MONASTERY: I don't believe in some-one being the Son of God or even God for that matter (forgive me if I'm wrong). So there's a hurdle there, but I always wanted to participate in one of those rituals with the smoke machines and sing in the same key as everyone else. Basically, I wanted to taste some faith.

2

Spirit Rock

My first journey was to Spirit Rock, considered the Mecca of mindfulness retreats. In the 1960s, a group of students looking for meaning dropped out of their Ivy League schools to go East and study Buddhism. Together they created mindfulness, making it accessible to those of us who don't speak Buddhist. They built Spirit Rock as well as several other retreats in the USA.

I thought I could deal with a month of mindfulness because I'd been practising it for around forty-five minutes a day for the last fifteen years, sitting in my closet with a lit candle under my statue of Buddha (so pretentious, but no one knows – well, you do now, but don't tell anyone). It's not easy being spiritual when you're sitting surrounded by your shoes and underwear, but it's all I've got. Ed wouldn't let me build a temple in the basement, so it's the closet. I thought, what's a month? I figured I'd end up either enlightened or insane.

1 February 2022

I entered the gates of Spirit Rock, a meditation retreat nestled in the middle of the curvy mountains of Marin County, above San Francisco. There wasn't a sign of civilization. Just those evergreens – so American, reaching to the heavens with hawks circling the highest branches and wild turkeys gobbling around the 200 acres. Paths squiggled up the hills through forests and streams, leading to log cabin dormitories with names like Loving-kindness, Equanimity, Compassion.

Mine was called Joy, which I hoped there would be some of because I had started to think maybe a month was too much. My room was about eight feet by twelve with a single bed. Folded top and bottom sheets and a pillowcase on top waiting for me to make it up. Ha ha! No chance! Until I remembered this was not a hotel, it was a monk's cell.

At 5.30pm after check-in, a loud gong rang. It scared me to death because the reverberations vibrate through every one of your organs. Your kidneys shake. Your uterus vibrates. This bell indicated we should all proceed to the main meditation hall.

The decor was very Zen: an inverted pyramid made of perfectly fitted planks of cedar. The floor area was afloat with zafus every few feet (they want it to sound spiritual, but it means cushions). There were small wooden tripods for people to perch on (like a proctologist would use), and piles of mats and foam of every size and shape to comfortably wedge between thighs and bottoms while sitting for the next 7,000 hours or whatever a month's worth of sitting is. I decided to sit on a chair and grabbed ten zafus, three blankets and four mats. I started hoarding to get ready to go to war with my mind.

There were about seventy of us and most everyone was in their twenties or thirties. How a twenty-year-old has the discipline to sit thirteen hours a day, I can't understand. At twenty, I had to be peeled off the ceiling, I was so wild. I know at past retreats I've been to (much shorter ones), the participants were older, clinging on to their hippie days:

Tibetan yak hats, smelling of patchouli oil and feet, draped in pendants of moons and angels, sometimes carrying a wand. All looking like aged warlocks and witches, which they probably were.

When I saw our schedule for the month I nearly bolted.

5.00am: Wake-up bell
5.30am – 6.30am: Meditate
6.30am – 8.00am: Breakfast
8.00am – 11.00am: Meditate
11.00am – 1.00pm: Lunch
1.00pm – 5.00pm: Meditate
5.00pm – 6.00pm: Tea
6.00pm – 7.00pm: Meditate
7.00pm – 8.15pm: Lecture
8.30pm – 9.00pm: Meditate
After 9.00 – For me a hospital

One of the teachers explained to us what mindfulness was in case any of the participants were stupid enough to sign up for a thirty-day retreat of doing something they've never heard of before. She set everyone straight. She said that mindfulness isn't about stopping thoughts but welcoming them all in without judging them. Thoughts are transient like weather patterns, constantly changing if you don't cling on to them and drum up a story. We would learn how to observe them rather than just obey them.

Another teacher (there were five) laid down the rules. She had a few feathers sticking out of her dreadlocks and a big tie-dye sack dress to hide whatever was going on under there. She also had that bad habit some meditation teachers have of speaking in that hushed, yogurty, dream-catchery tone as if her words were very precious and we should all be taking notes on her jewels of wisdom. Those people start all their sentences with 'So . . .' That's *so* irritating.

The rules were as follows. No intoxicants. No sex (like you could have it on your sliver of a bed). No killing anything, which is a let-down as it was on my to-do list, but I think they meant insects. They told us even if an ant is in your path, the rule is, walk around it, because it may have been your grandmother.

We did a little ritual, where we had to give our phones away to begin the cold turkey of coming off technology. We all had to queue up and one by one place our phones in a big bowl; each drop was accompanied by a reverberating gong on the Tibetan bowl. I panicked because I still had to make some urgent calls: order a bookshelf from Ikea, get some Chanel lipstick – urgent things. You got a little bow from the teachers when you finally released your phone. For days afterwards, I felt phantom vibrations and grabbed the air to connect to anyone.

The next thing on the agenda was we had to sign up for daily jobs. I made a beeline for the dishwashing team, thinking it was far better than loo duty.

Before the silence began, I was introduced to my three-person dishwashing team. A younger woman said to the man and me, 'Since you two are elders, why don't I take the difficult jobs and you do the easier ones?' How dare she address me as an elder? Luckily, they said no killing otherwise I would have gone for her throat. What is it about me that screams 'elder'? I didn't ask in case she came up with something, but I started the retreat completely bummed out.

A deafening gong announced the start of the retreat.

2 February 2022

As promised, at 5am, the Gong gonged. I didn't ever recollect seeing 5am in my life except after an all-nighter. As soon as I finally tore myself out of bed, I noticed that I had an insatiable itch on my back. I tried to get a look in the tiny mirror above the even tinier sink and there it was – a tumour: a large lump about an inch in height ending at a volcanic red tip. My first thought was I have cancer. I started smiling a little when I thought this might be my way out of Spirit Rock early with dignity.

Before leaving my room I tried to make my bed, which was the size of a sanitary towel. I couldn't get the sides even. I did this twelve more times and came to the conclusion that not only did I have cancer, I had OCD.

When I walked outside, in the sky I saw a gigantic white spotlight, bigger than all the other stars and about a quarter the size of the moon. It was as if a large truck with an ultra-bright headlight was heading towards me. I wanted to find out what it was, but I had no time to pursue it because I was dying.

I was too scared to sit and meditate with the lump on my back, thinking any moment it would burst and poison me, so I went to the office and asked them to find me a hospital and book me in fast. They looked at me in disgust because it was day one and already someone (me) was making trouble. I showed all of them the lump and as they gathered around, I could tell even they, the evolved office workers, found it gross. In America if you have insurance you can get instant help and if you don't, you're dead. If you have money you can also get heart surgery on the spot in seconds. Luckily, I had American insurance from when I lived there, so they could make an appointment for an immediate visit to a walk-in medical centre.

3 February 2022

I was so relieved I could talk on the way to the lump clinic. I gabbled away in fast speed to Phoenix (staff member, not the bird), who took me to the Carbon Health clinic in a shopping mall between Crate & Barrel and The Cheesecake Factory. You can order a lemon meringue straight from the surgery slab when you wake up. God forbid you stop eating for too long here in my country.

Missy, the receptionist, was wrapped in cellulite with beautiful American-flagged glitter fingernails clicking away on a keyboard. After filling in endless forms to find out how much money I had, I was met by a doctor who informed me I didn't have cancer even though the lump was now the size of a 36D bra cup. To cut a long story short, she lanced and drained it, all for the bargain basement price of a Tesla. I tried to stay in the mall by convincing Phoenix it was an emergency, that I had to get my legs shaved and buy popcorn in bulk. But Phoenix wasn't giving in and said, 'Get in the car.'

In a few hours, I was back at Spirit Rock, silent again. I did a day of practice, which ended at 9pm. When the Gong gonged to mark the session over, I realized I was asleep sitting up and snoring. I looked around in sheer panic to spot if anyone had noticed me. It was then I was smacked in the face with the reality that no one here was looking at me. They were not interested in me.

The fact that I was not the centre of the universe hit me hard. It looked like no one even cared, they were just in their own spiritual wombs. But to me, attention is the air I breathe. Without it, I don't exist. Which is why I entered the world of show business.

Before I left for Spirit Rock, friends of mine asked how I could go on a thirty-day silent retreat? I've done shorter retreats in the past. The silence is my favourite part. When you can nix the small talk while you're eating, you can actually taste food in all its delicious details. Usually, I just woof and while woofing, I'm getting ready for the next mouthful. But when you can concentrate on pure taste, you savour every tiny morsel of the granola. Other people around you are silent too, with eyes rolled back, hands clasping their hearts as they chew the cereal, worshipping the salty, sweet taste of cinnamon, molasses, dates with no one to interrupt their ecstasy with some mundane, 'What do you do?'

No, it wasn't the silence that was the hard part, it was the thirteen hours of doing mindfulness a day. As well as mindful sitting and mindful eating, we had mindful walking where you walk a distance of around fifteen feet very slowly, then turn and walk back. And then you repeat; back and forth. To an outsider, it would look fairly bizarre; more like a caged animal than an exercise to calm the mind. The idea is to feel every sensation of walking from placing the heel of the foot down, up to the toe and the sense of the foot leaving the ground, then the other leg swinging forward and placing the foot down, from heel to toe. When you lose focus because your thoughts have snared you again and carried you away to the past or future, you're meant to stop, and without any 'I've done it wrong' thinking, bring your focus back to where you last had it in your foot and then keep walking. This goes on for forty-five minutes about eight times a day, between all the forty-five minute 'sits'. If you don't lose your mind doing it, you might have accomplished what very few humans can do: to get your mind to kneel like you've just tamed a lion.

4 February 2022

The hair-raising Gong got me up at 5.00am, and as I woke I found I had shooting pains up my body and knew immediately I had polio. From my head to my toes, my nerves felt like lightning. I thought I couldn't go back to the office and say, 'Remember me? I was the one with cancer yesterday. Well, now I have polio. Can you help me?' I went into the office anyway and hunted for painkillers – I figured out you can't scream in silence – but all they had was hemp allergy salve and seaweed gum.

After lunch we had a break where we could do what we wanted except call, read, write or leave. I walked through the wooded forest and noticed it was getting harder and harder to move my limbs. With each leg weighing in at a ton and a half, I was thinking, 'I've whipped this body like an old plough horse for my whole life and now it's finally crumpling.' My body was saying, 'Haha, I've finally got your attention and now it's payback. You've abused me all these years with your high-speed jazzercise and extreme Zumba, and now I'm going to give you a taste of your own abuse.'

Suddenly I knew what it is to be old, and I thought this is how slowly I am going to walk for the rest of my life. My self-pity had gone off the charts. Tears in my eyes, I imagined myself walking towards my grave.

The disintegration of my body wasn't a complete fantasy. Twice a year I go to my doctor in London, who shoots a syringe full of something made from the coxcomb of a rooster into my knee. I kid you not. For those of you who don't know, the coxcomb is that red fleshy thing that hangs obscenely over on top of their heads. Yup, that's what ends up in my knees; to keep them young and springy. Without that juice, I've just got two bones grinding against each other.

As proof, earlier this year my doctor emailed me my 'prognosis'.

Prognosis of patient Ruby Wax:
Diagnosis: Bilateral knee osteoarthritis.
On examination, there are joint effusions with low-grade synovitis. She cannot achieve the last 5° of full extension. Flexion of the left knee is to 130° and flexion of the right knee is to 140°.
I have aspirated and injected both joints today, aspirating 20ml of non-inflammatory fluid and injecting 60mg of Depo-Medrone. I would like her to have updated X-rays. We feel that she is reaching the stage where she will need to see a knee surgeon to discuss the prospect of joint replacement surgery. The left knee is the more symptomatic.

I think this all means I'm fucked and will never skip again. So, there it was, proof that it wasn't my imagination. My body was deteriorating.

Buddha talked about death, and how transient our lives are, and now this was happening to me. I wonder if Buddha had knee problems, and if it motivated him to go through what he did?

6 February 2022

Tonight after dinner I went for my first night of dishwashing duty. I couldn't stand being cast in the role of 'the elder' by the younger dishwashing partner. I decided I would make her like me; make me her bestie. I wanted her to be aware of how well known I was in the UK rather than just being 'assistant' to Alpha dishwashing woman. She was doing the 'hard' job of rinsing and sponging the dirty dishes and then handing them to me, her second in command, to put the dishes into the appropriate slots on the rubber tray. The old man who really was an elder (unlike me) was ostracized. She sent him to the other side of the dishwashing machine, far away, to do menial, senile drying. We'd roll our eyes at each other whenever he made a mistake like dropping a cup, which meant he made even more mistakes. I was so happy he was screwing up and not me. I didn't want to be the victim. I know too well how it is to be treated like an ignorant lowlife.

Alpha girl was sponging dirty plates in Zen slow motion, showing the two of us how evolved she was. Trying to raise myself to her level, I also went into slo-mo Zen mode. Thich Nhat Hanh actually writes about mindful dishwashing. He says the idea is to become present. You should feel the plate in your hands, the warmth of the water, the smell of the soap, and the visuals of the bubbles. Thich says, 'Dishes themselves and the fact that I am here washing them are miracles! Each thought, each action in the sunlight of awareness becomes sacred. It may take a bit longer to do the dishes, but we can live fully, happily, in every moment.'

Well, that's what we did, sacredly washing and being one with each plate. It took hours. At the end, Alpha gave me a little Namaste bow acknowledging my good work. As we exited, we ignored the old man.

7 February 2022

I was walking on a path through the forest and ended up at a waterfall along the river. I noticed a plant with one very thin curly tendril and it reminded me of Sox with his one white eyebrow.

Only about a month ago my beloved cat died. Sox eventually grew to love me but for about fifteen out of his seventeen years he hated me. On the fifteenth, I broke him. From then on he'd sleep with me and let me pet him without trying to draw my blood. While I was on holiday in Cape Town, someone in London who was taking care of Sox said he had stopped eating, and that he was starting to look like a skeleton. A few days later she told me the vet said he had throat cancer. She said Sox was waiting to see me before he died. I didn't believe this hokum but when I finally came back to the UK, just an hour after I walked through the door, Sox began to make choking sounds. I howled like an animal all the way to the vet, who put him to sleep.

As I was saying, there was one white hair in Sox's eyebrow that stuck out, and it looked like that single curly tendril. And when I saw it that day at Spirit Rock, I felt the loss of my cat like a knife to my heart, and I completely broke down. When the Gong gonged, I dragged myself back to the meditation hall for the forty-five-minute sit, but I couldn't sit for long, I was too upset. I walked back to revisit Sox's memorial place.

On the way, I noticed my Tibetan hat on the path. I didn't even know I'd dropped it, that's how mindful I was. I put it back on and went to look for Sox's curly tendril. At the small stream, I decided to step down a few rocks to put my hand in the bubbling brook and feel the cold water. While I was climbing back up the three rocks, my knees gave out, I fell backwards and hit my head on the bottom rock. So, there I was lying head down in the river, partially under water. The only reason I didn't crack my head open was because I was wearing the Tibetan hat. (Buddha must have been watching.)

I scampered up quickly, looking around to see if anyone had seen the fall. I forgot no one sees me here. I walked back humiliated and shaking, then I realized I had sprained my thumb. On top of the cancer and polio, now my hand had to be wrapped in an ice pack in the office. I was sure people were looking at me as if I was a sad old loser. I could hear my dad's voice telling me how everything I do is a screw-up. He used to say, 'Oh boy, now you're in trouble big time. There's one rule for everybody and another for Ruby Wax. Who do you think you are, a Princess? You're pathetic. Always the one not fitting in. Always, the troublemaker.'

That evening, I was scared I'd lose my dishwashing place and the old guy would take over my job, so even though I was in pain I went into the kitchen to wash plates. I didn't want Alpha girl to think I was a wimp. I kept my position and silently showed her my bruised thumb. She bowed at the end of our washing session, acknowledging my bravery.

10 or 15 February 2022?

I don't have my phone so I don't really know what day it is. I just made that up. I signed up to be the gonger at the 3pm sit.

There were volunteers throughout the day to sit in front of the meditation group and they had to gong when the forty-five minutes were up.

So, I was in charge of the 3pm gonging, and I noticed that not many people had shown up to my session. Of course, I took it personally. I got the heart-sinking sadness I used to feel when doing matinées of my one-woman show to an almost empty theatre. I'd actually count the empty seats, and I'd feel my heart ache so much I could hardly do the show. I was that upset. Rather than thinking people who had bought tickets were ill or had some other important reason they couldn't come, I assumed they hated me and I would be almost as disappointed in myself as my father was.

The thin crowd of meditators sat before me cross-legged on their mountain of cushions. They all had their eyes shut and this hit another trigger in me: they didn't want to even look at me. I knew they were meditating, but I couldn't help feeling the familiar burn of neglect. My instinct was to say some funny lines from my comedy show so they'd realize I was very talented and not just a person who gongs at the end of sitting.

I gazed at all the beautiful boys sitting serenely in a cloud of calm, wrapped in their sacred shawls. I kept my eyes lowered, not wanting them to catch that I was gawking at them like an old perv. When the forty-five minutes passed and I gonged the Gong (rather well, I thought), everyone who'd been sitting stood up and did the traditional bow. I pretended the bow was to me personally for doing a great show. In reality there are Buddha statues at the back of the platform I was sitting on and after every sitting everyone gives them a bow. But I took the fantasized personal acclaim anyway, and when I left, I was still waiting to be asked for an autograph.

10 February 2022

Last night I found a calendar in the garbage. I know what day it is again. The turkeys had a cat fight this morning. I watched two males in a fight to the death over a female. I interpreted this dance as, 'Don't try and fuck with my womenfolk.' They were doing a face-off, with their tail feathers fanned out and their legs lifting and claws high, like they were doing a slow-motion German march. They had started hissing, and one of them went for the neck of the other and 'bang bang banged' his body back and forth, whacking him on the ground until there was just a heap of feathers. What was left of the defeated and nearly bald turkey was then chased off the hill. The bald bird loser had to walk the walk of shame into the forest in disgrace and I know will be ostracized forever. I know how humiliated he feels. Nature can be so cruel.

I watched the hawks circling in the sky and was so moved by their streamlined grace, and then noticed they were circling because they were waiting for something to die so they could peck it to death. So much for care in the community.

There's nothing to do at Spirit Rock, nowhere to go, nothing to buy. Your thoughts can't grab on to anything. But I badly needed to do something, so I went on a search for the perfect rock which, in my mind, was evenly round and smooth. When I found one, I took it to my room. The next day, I noticed its imperfections, and I wasn't happy with it. I returned, threw it back among the other rocks and looked around for a more perfect rock. Going shopping, then returning the item the next day, is something I love to do. I thought, 'Desperate times.'

At this point about ten days in, my thoughts started to give up their internal tirades. They didn't shut off completely, but they became more like fireworks that are losing their fizz mid-flight. I'd think things like, 'You forgot to buy . . .' (I'd forget what I had to buy), 'You have to call . . .' (I'd have no idea who).

I walked up to the top of the hill to what I called 'my chair'. I used to get pissed off when I'd find other people sitting on 'my chair'. I wondered where I got the idea that it was mine? I started to notice how crazy these kinds of thoughts were. How big was my ego to think public furniture was mine?

There was a Buddha statue in front of 'my tree', where I watched a lizard leap around Buddha's face and then go stock still on his forehead. I thought there was a lesson there, that even if you're Buddha, a lizard can still sit on your face. I found that comforting.

That afternoon, I watched tiny moving dots on the ridge on the high mountain that faced me across the valley. It gradually occurred to me that those dots were people walking along the top. Immediately I got that burning envy that I should be up there. I wanted to spring off my chair and run straight up that mountain, to show those people I was no slouch; I was an athlete. Then it struck me with heart-pinching agony that I couldn't run up, let alone walk up, because of the arthritic knees. That didn't stop me. To prove to myself that I still had it, I decided to run down the hill, along an uneven pathway through the forest to ground level. The result was when I got to the bottom, I couldn't move. My legs were in spasm and I needed to lie on a bench. For the rest of the day, I hated myself for being old and inept.

12 February 2022

Something strange has happened. In my mind, I've started to assign the people on the retreat roles as if they were characters in a play I'd written. I cast them based on who they reminded me of. It struck me that I do this in real life: projecting personalities on people I have never met before. All my first impressions and probably all impressions are biased judgements and wild guesses about who they really are. Quickly assessing, are they friend or foe? Smart or stupid? Cruel or kind? I'm like an omnipotent casting director.

There was a woman sitting behind me in the meditation hall with Janis Joplin-like neurotic hair, extra wide child-bearing hips and the hands of a peasant who's been working the soil for fifty years. I cast her as an Earth Mother who would protect me from harm, especially from dangerous men. Because she was behind me, I thought she literally had my back: she was the mother I should have had.

I got it into my head that the young blond guy who was my permanent neighbour on my right had a crush on me, and was sneaking looks at me when I had my eyes shut. I used to watch him out of the corner of my eye to see if I could catch him, but I never did, mainly because he wasn't looking at me. Then I'd be hurt, feeling abandoned by someone who didn't even know I existed. How crazy is that? He reminded me of a boy I stalked when I was about fourteen years old. I was heartbroken that my high-school crush never phoned or sent me a Valentine's Day card. How could he? I'd never met the guy. I'd tailed him down the hallway, sneaking behind pillars and peeping out so he wouldn't catch me. My best friend at the time finally nabbed him and lost her virginity to him. I never spoke to her again, but I did send her a greeting card that had written on it, 'Congratulations on your grand opening!' What are the chances of finding a card with that on it?

13 February 2022

Of the five teachers who gave talks a few times a week, we were each assigned to one for personal sessions. We'd meet with them every other day. I think the idea was to keep an eye on us in case we lost our minds rather than found them. These private meetings were the only time we were allowed to speak. I'll call my teacher T.

T looked like a big charismatic red-faced stand-up comic. His delivery often had me laughing and then I'd realize he was serious, but just when he'd convince me he was serious, he'd twinkle to indicate it was a joke. I loved him even more because he was slightly camp. I love that in a Buddhist.

R: *I hurt all over, it's happening every day now.*

T: *Where is the pain exactly?*

R: *It's moving around. One minute it feels like I'm being stabbed in the right side of my back, then it stops and moves to the left. Same with my neck. Then it feels like I might have polio, then cancer, then a heart attack. The pain is switching on and off like electricity all around my body. Luckily I can walk slowly without feeling like an old person, because everyone is walking slowly; the* *younger, the slower. So at least I'm not ashamed about being decrepit because no one can tell.*

T: *Listen to what your body is telling you. Try to experience it from the inside.*

R: *Feeling inside your body? Is that what they mean when they say embodiment? I thought it was like what they wrap a mummy in?*

T: *It means you're aware of the sensations rather than just living in your head. You should go through your body section by section and listen out for what it wants you to know. You probably haven't paid that kind of attention to your body before.*

R: *It's taken its revenge. Why should I pay attention to it when it's letting me down everywhere I look. Each day, a droop there, a new hair here.*

T: *Maybe it knows you're not happy with it. So many people want their bodies to be perfect. They clench them to make themselves look slimmer, creating tension in the muscles and making the bones rigid.*

R: *Today I got mad at it just because I couldn't zip up my fly, talk about letting myself down.*

T: *You should honour this body of yours. If you think about how it was formed, it's a miracle. I mean our teeth are made of calcium which came from stars exploding. Our biology, the chemicals in us, are all a result of the Big Bang.*

R: *And here we are, treating them like some old golf cart that moves our heads from place to place. I wasn't aware I was related to the Big Bang. What else?*

T: *Your mind leaves you all the time, wandering this way and that, your body never leaves you except when you die.*

R: *So how do I show my body that I care, especially after it's given me so much grief?*

T: *Rather than live in your head, experience things directly. When you hear something, focus on hearing it, or when you smell something, focus on the details of the smell, same with seeing something. This direct experience is what being present is all about, and when you're present there's no clenching or thinking what's wrong with you. You're just sensing, not thinking. It relaxes you and you're awake for the journey.*

I want to give you this poem to read when you have time.

I read it before I went to bed.

> If you find yourself half naked
> And barefoot in the frosty grass, hearing
> Again, the earth's great sonorous moan that says
> You are the air of the now and gone, that says
> All you love will turn to dust,
> And will meet you there, do not
> Raise your fist. Do not raise
> Your small voice against it. And do not
> Take cover. Instead, curl your toes
> Into the grass, watch the cloud
> Ascending from your lips. Walk
> Through the gardener's dormant splendour
> Say only, Thank you
> Thank you.

 er reading it I wanted to give BAFTAs to all my limbs.

15 February 2022

Another meeting with T.

R: *I loved your poem. It almost made me cry but I can't because I'm taking so much medication.*

T: *When you feel you love something, enjoy every second of feeling it. Don't try to hold on too tightly because then you're chasing for more. Just think whatever arises also passes.*

R: *I should be thinking of those types of things. I'm sitting here thirteen hours a day and usually I'm thinking of something incredibly vacuous like what are the lyrics of that song Phoebe sings in Friends? 'Something, something smelly cat . . .?' I don't want to think about things like arising and passing. It makes me think about ageing. I'm so ashamed about my age, it seems like a failure on my part. My mother was so ashamed of her age, she'd tell people she was my sister.*

T: *You can be young at seventy-nine and old at nineteen, depending on how flexible a mind you have. If you keep your viewfinder open and are curious about how other people see the world, that's a young mind. If you think how you see the world is how everyone should see it, it's an old mind. You're only as old as your mind is.*

R: *Is that supposed to make me feel better? That my body is crumbling but my mind is a young whippersnapper?*

16 February 2022

While I was doing my dish duty – being handed plates by Alpha and slotting them into the tray – I got this idea which I thought was inspired. I walked out of the washing area into the dining room and began to take dirty plates directly from people who were about to put them in the soaking tubs full of water. I'm sure it had never been done before. It was like offering valet service for dishes. After taking the plate from their hands, I would pass it to Alpha girl through the opening to the kitchen. When I took their plates, the people gave me little bows of appreciation with their hands in Namaste position. Well, can you imagine how much my ego was fed? I got a bow, and I didn't even have to do a show! I just took a plate and bowed back. To be honest, I was slightly disgusted by how I always have to find the spotlight.

17 February 2022

I was looking out the window when I was supposed to be meditating (this happens a lot) and my mind had flown continents away. Then I caught sight of the turkeys. Instant happiness! Forgetting all about mindfulness, I began thinking what a great life turkeys must have right up until Thanksgiving rolls around. But even when it does, they have no idea about the holiday or date and what's going to happen to them. (I beg anyone reading this to please change your menu at Thanksgiving, I don't care what you eat but not turkeys. To me, at this moment, they are the most beautiful animal on the planet.)

Now I've really lost myself in thought; meditation out the window. I'm thinking about how lucky animals and insects are not knowing they're going to die. I'm thinking now of male spiders who insist on mating even though right afterwards they'll get their heads chewed off by the female. Every time! They never learn the lesson and maybe if they did know, they'd never believe it. It's not that different for people in some ways, they don't learn either. I know lots of women who'll always be attracted to the same type of man and then be surprised when they get dumped after they've had sex. I know it's not like getting your head chewed off but still, it's something to think about, which I shouldn't be because I'm doing mindfulness and should be focused on my breath. Okay, I'm aware my mind derailed and that counts as being mindful. I'm still trying to remember those lyrics of 'Smelly Cat'. What's wrong with me? My brain has gone to Comedy Central.

18 February 2022

The next day, at my private meeting with T, I brought up the idea of wanting to be happy.

R: *Isn't that what we're all doing here? Finding happiness? I mean isn't that why we're sitting here a hundred hours a day?*

T: *I think having the experience of happiness should come out of left field. If you chase it, you'll never find it.*

R: *Please don't tell me to think positive. I hate those people who tell you to think positively, it makes me feel like I'm even more of a failure.*

T: *Don't beat yourself up. Instead of trying to think positive, try to bring an image into your mind that gives you joy.*

R: *When I try to think about joy, I can only think about my cat, Sox, and then I remember he just died so I get even more depressed.*

That night I pictured Sox in my mind to try to bring up a positive feeling. It hurt my heart but underneath it felt like that tingly thing which I associate with love. I was so stunned I could switch on that tingly thing.

19 February 2022

I got up today at 4am before anyone else. That wasn't me in my real life but I wanted to experience just once what outside was like at that time, before the Gong, when no one else was awake. I opened the dorm door and stepped out.

It was like falling into Outer Space. I've never heard Nothing before. It was as if the world got soundproofed. The ground was glittering under the lamps. Everything was perfect and where it should be, even me. I felt like I had finally come home. I was just right there and sensed everything. I heard the snow moving, my breathing and silence. When the first Gong of the day gonged, I heard footsteps and with a heavy heart I knew I wasn't alone any more.

Gravity had returned. I could still see that white blinding spotlight in the sky, the same one I see every night and early morning. I had thought when it was just hovering above the cliffs, it was a drone that lit up so planes didn't fly into the mountains. What confused me was that tonight the round light was almost next to the moon, so how could it be a drone that high up? It looked like what I imagine a UFO looks like but if it was, I'm sure someone would break their silence and mention it.

I left the first 'sit' early so I could hear the gobble of turkeys, which always made my heart leap. That sound automatically switched on happiness in me and I was trying to memorize the feeling inside, to 'embody' it. See, I was picking up the lingo? I stood there, alone and smiling. As I ran towards the gobble sounds so as to not miss a single one, I was hit by a celestial chorus of starlings, operatically calling to each other. Because I was surrounded by a ring of tall mountains, the sound echoed. Miles and miles of sounds circling me. It was like I was in the middle of a whirlpool of starlings gossiping. The birds landed on trees simultaneously, filling every branch as if knowing instinctively how to decorate a Christmas tree. When they took off all at once, they filled the sky with hieroglyphic patterns. How do they know how to do synchronized flying without bumping into each other?

Suddenly a small dark frisbee crossed my path. Then another frisbee, and another one. I realized the turkeys were launching themselves from the hillside where they slept in the forest. When they first wake up (pre-gobble) they sound like demented evil witch children. When they wake up, they start hurtling themselves in an out-of-control arch across the walkway. One by one, it was like each turkey was being fired from a cannon and ended up splatted awkwardly on the frozen ground where they began their chorus of gobbles.

21 February 2022

It was T's turn to give the talk this evening. T spoke about how we're always 'streaming', not to do with television, but with our lives. He uses the term 'streaming' because he used to canoe when he was young. He thought streaming was a good metaphor for how he had to navigate along a stream, comparing it to the current that runs through our lives. The canoe and our lives never stop moving, he said. In canoeing terms, we need to learn when it's time to let the stream carry us – he called this 'flowing' – and when to take control by using the paddle to steer us around the rocks. He called that 'knowing'.

He said, if we try for too much control, fighting against the current, we exhaust ourselves, but if we let go too much, we might go out of control or tip over.

Applied to life, flowing means just taking your hands off the controls and knowing means being aware of what's going on. In order to live with ease, we have to balance both of those. Streaming, he said, also means being aware that everything arises and passes. Nothing arises unless something passes. If you don't breathe in you won't breathe out. Nothing is born if something doesn't die. Once the idea becomes embedded, he told us, even when something terrible happens, you know it will pass.

According to T, people create a reality that they believe is permanent, and dedicate their lives to avoid noticing change. Change will happen. Like it or not, here it comes. Our skin sheds and a whole new army of cells are born to keep us held in that casing known as 'you', but outside of that we're in a constant state of flux. We're always streaming. Nothing stays static – though you may think you can grab on to time and keep it still, it will drag you through your life screaming and kicking.

24 February 2022

I woke up at 4am again and rushed out into the night or morning or whatever it was. It's become my favourite time.

When I opened the dorm door, I just stood frozen in a state of wonder. I thought, 'Ruby, it's amazing, you're "present" right Now. Call Eckhart Tolle and tell him.' Then all my senses suddenly switched on at once at high volume. I could focus on the tiny detail of everything I heard, saw, smelled, and touched. I thought, I've either gone mad or I'm enlightened. I stared for I didn't know how long, at lattices of crystals. Each snowflake was made out of spiderweb-thin icicles; all of them had perfect geometry. They glittered like diamonds. I loved everything in that moment. I loved my hard bed with its one dingy blanket. I loved my dollhouse sink. I loved the heater I stole from someone's room. I loved the bathroom I had to share with everyone on my floor. And the turkeys and I were practically engaged.

25 February 2022

Tonight another teacher, D, spoke about what she called 'The thread of harm'.

She told us about growing up in an abusive family, and how as an adult she was aggressive, mainly to bring people under her control so they wouldn't hurt her first. She used to abuse her staff. As a lawyer, her aggression made her a success but a nightmare as a coworker. She terrorized her kids too, but until one of them pointed it out, she had no idea of the frightening effect she had on people.

D pointed out that 'a thread of harm' runs through all of us, and that we need to identify what it is before we can rid ourselves of it. That hit a big home run for me. I've been told I sometimes scare people. If I'm honest, it hasn't always been unconscious, I've done it on purpose to weaken the other person. I do that so I don't feel I'm the weak and helpless one. When I believe someone's not using their brain, or doesn't even have a brain, and is screwing up something that means a lot to me, I'll make a cutting remark and then smile, which confuses them, so they'll probably screw up even more, or say something even more stupid. Then I'll take another swipe at my prey. I'll say something confrontational and then I'll smile again, at which point they'll feel deflated, and they won't even realize why. I'm not proud of this repulsive habit, but I picked it up from Daddy when he played his games of cat and mouse with me. D said to break this habit, we should observe our urge to do harm before we act on it.

I fell asleep after the late evening meditation. Amazing how sitting in silence can be so exhausting. So many nights after the last sit I've found myself waking with a snort, and I sit up, expecting everyone will be staring at me. They never are.

Even though we never speak or look at each other, there's a feeling that we're all connected. Bonded in silence. Everyone is genuinely kind to each other. When you walk into a room, the person in front of you always holds the door open. If someone wants salt, everyone at the dinner table is so tuned in, someone will intuitively know to pass it.

It was at this point in the retreat, I noticed my mind was steady. There was so much free space in there, I could focus on snails making their slimy way up a branch or listen to frogs croaking for several hours. There was nowhere to go and nothing to do and that was fine with me. I'd notice people standing stock still, riveted on an ant's journey up a tree and then back down again. And of course, I was always up for turkey time. If I heard a gobble, I'd run to the sound and bathe in pure joy.

26 February 2022

One morning, I had the strangest experience. I couldn't tell if I was sleeping or awake, but when the Gong gonged, I felt completely unhurried and at ease. (This never happens.) My thoughts were so quiet they were more like a faint breeze inside my head. The demonic captain of the ship had jumped overboard, and I was left alone and at peace. There was no tension, no stress. It felt as if Sox was alive and well and living in me. My skin inside felt like it was lined with fur. I knew that if I consciously tried to stay in this state, I would break the spell, but in that moment I could feel everything in minute detail: the sheet on my body; the shifting of one foot and then the other; the breath moving in and out of my lungs.

I walked from the dorm to the café in that state; awake to everything in sight and alert to every sound. As I reached the bottom of the slope, I felt the feelings flow out of me as mysteriously as they came in. So many hours of sitting for so many days was worth it for those three or four minutes.

I met with T later that day.

R: *I think I may have been enlightened.*

T: *(Laughs) I once thought that happened to me and it was so thrilling, I went on to become a monk in Burma just to capture that feeling again. I never got it back. I tried so hard to become the perfect meditator that I got ill from over-exhaustion, and eventually had to give back the robes. I wasn't paying attention to what my body needed so it collapsed on me, I made it sit for hours, deprived it of sleep and ate badly.*

R: *Sometimes I wish I never started meditating because it makes me more aware of when I'm over-thinking. Then I start over-thinking about how I shouldn't be over-thinking.*

T: *Yeah, tell me about it.*

When I left his room, I looked up at the sky; the clouds were in the shape of an angel which turned into a dragon and then back into an angel. It made me think how everything is always transforming and I have absolutely no control over it. It struck me that I was having a thrilling rather than a frightening thought for a change.

27 February 2022

It was our second to last day and everything had transformed. I now loved everyone without exception, even the people I used to hate. Really loved them. I loved the woman who'd been getting on my nerves since day one. She always nabbed the seat by the window in the dining room to get the best view of the turkeys. I once took her seat and thought I saw her 'huffing' at me, so I made up a whole story about how she had personal problems. I also hated that she always dressed in purple.

I now loved the woman who had sat in front of me (I only saw the back of her head) in the meditation hall. She always nodded and did a little all-knowing guffaw when one of the teachers said something spiritual-sounding to show us all that she, and she alone, had a personal relationship with Buddha.

I realized that I'd got all these people wrong. We were all just humans trying to find some peace. We were connected like all those snowflakes were connected.

28 February 2022 – the last day

That last morning when we all lined up to get our phones back, I didn't want to ever see mine again. (This feeling passed an hour out of the retreat.) After the ceremony of giving back the phones we were allowed to speak again. I watched how I moved among people, making connections, checking out who was the most popular and wanting their approval. But this time I was more awake to my old habits.

I continued observing how wrong I'd been in my judgement of people. For the last month I'd been watching this overly large guy in the dining room, who ate with his mouth open. It drove me crazy how he would go back for second and third helpings. (I did that too.) I assumed he was going to be slow-witted. But when we finally spoke, I found out he had a great sense of humour. Far from being unintelligent, he was president of his own drug firm.

I had assumed a fellow member of the Turkey Fan Club was a redneck from down South on the basis of the fact she wore dowdy overalls, working men's boots and had a kerchief around her neck. Turns out she's the international director of a department for abused women as part of Médecins Sans Frontières (Doctors Without Borders). She's also a doctor who flies around the world to war-torn countries and saves lives.

And the man I assumed was a serial killer was a Harvard Professor in astrophysics.

The teachers offered advice on how to deal with going back into our lives. They said, 'If your friends ask what it was like here, you may want to just answer, "Okay." It's hard to describe an experience like this. It's an internal journey, so words may not be able to convey anything.' She's right, I thought. What would I say? 'I sat and followed my breath for thirty days?'

We took a tea break. I saw there was a note for me on the noticeboard. Each day, hoping to break the monotony of sitting and walking, we'd gathered around the message board to see if anyone had messaged us. Some lucky people received notes but I had never scored one of those folded pieces of paper with my name on it. Today, I was Mrs Lucky. There it was: a small piece of paper with my name on it. It said I should go to the office.

The office staff, whom I now also loved, told me I'd had an urgent email which they had printed out for me. The email was from my agent. It said that I had been offered an ad for potato chips. It was scheduled to shoot on Monday morning, the day after I got back. Since she couldn't reach me, and it was a very lucrative offer, she had accepted it on my behalf.

My immediate reaction was to email back and turn it down so as not to ruin this hard-earned month of disciplining my mind, but the word 'lucrative' made me hesitate. I could feel my cathedral of peace beginning to collapse.

Once we returned from the tea break, one of the teachers invited us to ask her questions if we wanted. By now I was dizzy with confusion. I raised my hand immediately and asked for advice about what I should do. She told me that after a long retreat, I should be alone and quiet for at least a week. I lied: I told her I had to accept the job or I'd be sued because I'd signed a contract (I hadn't). As an alternative, she advised me to treat the job as another mindfulness exercise: to remember when I felt the pressure mounting, to focus on my body, follow my breath, tune into sounds, feel the chair under me. Anything physical that would stop the thoughts from spiralling.

I went back to the office and emailed my agent to say 'yes' to the potato crisp job. She wrote back quickly, asking if I would mind starting my book tour the same night. I thought, well, I'm fairly evolved at this point, I can handle it. I went back into the hall and now my mind was filling up again with an internal argument about should I cancel the potato crisp ad and stay pure, or take the money and run? Guess which way I went?

There was a final exercise. It was designed to bring us back to the real world, and to help us communicate better with other people. We were instructed to find a partner and one of us had to speak for three minutes about how this experience had changed us and then we'd change roles. When I spoke, my voice was a croak, like I'd smoked 10,000 cigarettes. I was shocked as I observed myself trying to be funny to get the other person to like me. But I held back, wanting to speak from the heart, not the mind. I tried to listen when my partner spoke, rather than think about what I would say next. My partner was as gentle with me as I was to her. There was a sweetness that passed between us.

At the end of this exercise, we were told to strip our beds and make them up for the next retreat which was due to start in two hours. That was a rude awakening. See how disposable we are? Everything arises and passes, especially us.

I left Spirit Rock hugging everyone and blubbering how much I loved them, even though I never spoke to them. In a state of utter desolation, I said goodbye to each turkey, promising them I'd come back to them next year. They pecked as usual, but I think it meant goodbye.

The shuttle was coming in about ten minutes, but I had to say goodbye to my favourite spot on top of the mountain where I'd watch the hawks circling and the lizard crawling on the Buddha's head. At 'my chair', I wept that I wouldn't see it again. Because I was so carried away by the beauty of it all, when I got back down I was told the first shuttle had left. I heard my dad say, 'There's one rule for everyone and another one for Ruby Wax.' But I didn't care any more. I had my own rules. I was so calm, I just waited for the next shuttle.

I shared the car with the boy I thought had a crush on me. I introduced myself as the woman who sat next to him in the hall for the last thirty days. I asked if he ever noticed me and if he did, what did he think was going on in my head? He said he never noticed me. So much for four weeks of courtship. The shuttle dropped me off at the airport and being hit by the noises of real life nearly burst my eardrums.

When you begin to move in the real world again, you're slightly shaky. You're like a new-born colt, scrawny and weak on their bendy stick legs that keep collapsing under them. I boarded the plane in this colt-like condition. When I asked the woman in the seat next to me if there was anything going on in the world that I should know about, she said, 'Yes, there's a war on.'

Oh, by the way, do you remember I spoke about seeing a bright blinding light every night in different positions in the sky? Are you still wondering what it was? When we could finally speak again, someone at the retreat told me it was Venus. And when the sun came up on the other side of the sky, it disappeared from the shadow of the earth. I was so relieved, I thought it had been a UFO.

Clinic

16 May 2022

BANG!! BANG!! BANG!! BANG!!

I'm at my fifth rTMS session and it seems to be accelerating on the pain and noise front. The guy who's in charge of the procedure is moving the dial up from 40 to 42. That may not sound a lot to you, but the intensity goes from fast skull hammering to it sounding like someone is drilling into cement to break up the sidewalk; I am the sidewalk. I suppose it's better than what they used to do to mentally ill people in the old days. They'd put them in a swing and whizz them around for hours or lock them in freezing baths. They claimed these procedures were cures, but really they were punishing patients for having mental issues. Starting in the seventeenth century, people who behaved too bizarrely were burnt at the stake, probably being mistaken for witches. So I'm lucky I'm just getting hammered.

Just like at Spirit Rock, almost everyone at the mental clinic is in their twenties and thirties. I don't know why that happened. Did all the old people die? I miss the older crazies. I fondly remember one ancient woman who actually lived in the mental ward asking me, 'Why is there a dentist living in my back molar?' Those were the days.

There are things to be grateful for; in a mental clinic no one has FOMO. You might see someone who's young and gorgeous, but behind closed doors she's probably eating the wallpaper.

Shrink session

R: *Why do you think I ganged up on the old guy with this woman? I didn't even like her.*

S: *This is exactly what you did in the past. It was your survival tactic.*

R: *What tactic am I using from my past?*

S: *You colluded with a woman you thought was powerful enough to protect you from your father.*

R: *We ganged up on the older guy because he was like my dad? And she was helping me kick the shit out of him?*

S: *It's very hard to let go of something that made you feel safe as a girl, even though you don't need it in the present.*

R: *My father shows up everywhere. He never washed a dish in his life.*

*

I passed the test that proves I'm not suicidal, so I'm going to be one of the lucky people who's allowed out. Today I have my first visitor. A nurse comes into my room and tells me there is a guest waiting for me. They won't allow anyone to come upstairs in case they report back that the ward looks like a dust bowl. Also, it probably wouldn't be a good idea for them to see Zombie girl with the chewed-off teddy bear head. So, we meet downstairs. (No elevator.)

I see the look on my friend's face when she sees me. She tries to tell me I look fine. I know I look like I've been in a dishwasher for a year.

If I was on the addiction or anorexic ward and I tried to walk out the front entrance, there'd be an eardrum-shattering alarm, and the sound of running feet, and security would fling me back in. But no, after a phone call to confirm that I am not about to self-harm or harm someone else, the doors fly open. My friend and I only make it to the corner before I have to turn back. There's too much reality outside.

17 May 2022

The next day another friend comes to see me. While we wait for the phone call to confirm I've been given permission to leave, I pretend to pull out the drinking fountain from the floor. You know, like the Native American chief in *One Flew Over the Cuckoo's Nest*. No one thinks I'm funny.

As the doors open, I shout, 'Elvis is leaving the building.' They don't find this funny either.

We walk outside and I'm clutching my friend's arm like a very old woman. Everything is too loud. She walks me to her house – I'm making slow progress – which is around the corner. At least the house is familiar territory, and just sitting there within its four solid walls, I feel safe. I can't sit there for very long though, so she shuffles me back to the clinic. I go straight to bed. I'm exhausted and the sleeping pills are delicious.

18 May 2022

A and F came to take me out. We went to a park. I thought I was acting normal but once in a while I'd see them look at each other like, 'What happened to her?' They delivered me back to the safety of the clinic. I always feel relieved when those doors swing open and let me back in.

20 May 2022

More people are coming to take me out for walks. I think I'm in too much pain to have visitors. I'm constantly feeling I have to put on a show, so I pitch my voice up higher and smile-jerk my face to look like I'm happy.

Sometimes we go to the park. I still don't feel connected to the real world, but I enjoy watching the swans, and I'm able to see happy people crossing the lawn without wanting to kill them. They're not talking about how sick they are, but I find that's all I can talk about. What else is there?

When friends first started phoning me, I was so excited, I made a schedule in my notebook of who I'd like to see and when. Sometimes there were three different sets of people coming in a single day. Then I realized this was insane behaviour. I was ill. So I crossed everyone's name out, and turned off my phone.

22 May 2022

I decided I can only handle family coming from now on. It's too much effort to do so much acting. Ed and I go to the hotel next door for tea. It's sort of Ritz-ish. There's someone plinking on a grand piano and silver service scones and tea are served by servile bow-tied waiters. There are palms throughout and chandeliers drip from the mile-high glass ceilings. I can spot horror on the maître d's face when he sees me. I'm wearing a coat over pyjamas with oiled sticky-up hair. He walks us quickly to an alcove behind a cluster of palms. I think it's because he recognizes me from TV and he wants to protect my privacy as I'm an important VIP. Then I figure out it's to hide me from the public and I'm bringing down the place a hundred notches.

3

Humpbacks

Ring the bells that still can ring,
Forget your perfect offering, There's a crack in everything,
That's how the light gets in.

– Leonard Cohen

In those last days at Spirit Rock, my thoughts were more peaceful than painful. What a change! If I had to sit for thirty days for a state of mind like that, I'd do it again.

When I flew home from San Francisco, my mind was a joy to live in. My internal weather condition was sunny with a slight breeze and no clouds. It was just big open-hearted country. Even when I was sitting on the plane I felt fine, and I'm terrified of flying. One bump and I'm clawing the ceiling. But this time I had no fear, just a warm tingling in my heart. That 'Sox' feeling again.

1 March 2022

I landed in Heathrow in a blissful condition. In the Uber, I was still blissful. When I got home, I wasn't so blissful any more. I just stood there in the kitchen waiting for instructions. I missed the routine of knowing whether I should sit, or walk, or if it was time for lunch. I missed the sound of the Gong.

Suddenly five minutes in, my phone was gang-banging me with messages about tomorrow's shoot. There were missed calls from the makeup artist, director, producer, script writer, stylist; there were pick-up times and drop-off times for the following day. I could feel the new nicer, calmer me being shoved aside, and something more bristly stepping in.

To block out the reality of what was waiting to devour me next day, I turned on the television like an old junkie going back to her drug of choice. I've always used television to distract myself from my demons, either watching it or being on it.

Every channel was showing outlines of maps on the screen indicating chunks of land that had been devoured by Russian troops. I remembered being told there was a war in Ukraine. I was staring at coloured areas on a map representing the Apocalypse. They showed various cities and towns, and I stood, breathing in the horror. My blissful feeling had left the building.

Usually, I try to avoid the news. Just hearing the theme of the BBC News, with those foreboding trumpets and the beating drums getting you ready to 'Charge!' – followed by the sound of 'beep beep beeeeeeeeep' like the world has just 'flatlined' – is warning enough to make me turn the TV off. The BBC played that horror show recording before their daily listing of how many people died from Covid. They might as well have played that old Black Death favourite, 'Bring out your dead'. If it had been available in Shakespeare's time, that terror-evoking orchestration is what Henry the Fifth would have used for background music when he addressed the soldiers. He would have stood there on the breach in his full hose and jerkin, his sword drawn, and 'beep beep beep' sounds running underneath his speech (the speech that starts with 'Once more unto the breach, dear friends, once more . . . But when the blast of war blows in our ears . . . Stiffen the sinews, summon up the blood.' (Shakespeare wrote that. Did you think I did?)

So here I was, an hour after getting home, with my nose pressed to the TV screen and panicking as I watched the unreal but all-too-real footage of people who had been crushed under their homes and were being dug out. Other people were walking in shock. I saw old people with tears, hundreds of rivulets, dripping down their cheeks. From the lack of expression on their cracked and bereaved faces, it appeared to me they had given up. Entire families who looked like ours, kids who dressed like our kids, clutching their confused pets, walked over a plank of wood they used as a bridge over the flood from an exploded sewer.

And what was happening in my life? Well, I had a potato chip ad scheduled for the next morning, so I dyed my hair!

At Spirit Rock I didn't give a shit what I looked like. I'd never looked in a mirror, but now that I had, I saw there was an out-of-control wheat field growing out of me. So I removed all my body hair (like anyone would notice when they watched the ad).

When Ed came home at the end of the day there was no time to talk because a car had arrived to take me into the city. Since there was a 6am hair and makeup call, the producer had decided it would be a good idea if I stayed overnight in a hotel close to the shooting location.

I had no idea this hotel existed. It was squished between two glass and steel monoliths in the London Bridge area. It was probably the weirdest hotel on the planet. On the outside it resembled a simple Georgian house; on the inside it looked more like a cross between the Taj Mahal and a toilet.

Titanic-sized rooms were coated in purple velvet. Numerous gigantic chandeliers were hanging above. Several paintings of the rich, pockmarked hotel owner (not a beauty) were hanging in plastic gold frames covered in a sprinkling of dust. It was India's answer to *The Shining*.

I was informed the restaurant was closed, so I went out into the rainy night of London to find something to eat. Nothing was open. Now I know there's a war in Ukraine but I was hungry and irritated; so much for the compassion training.

2 March 2022

It was still raining when I walked out of the hotel early next morning to look for a taxi. There were none. In London, taxis don't like to get wet. After eventually locating a passing taxi, I hurled myself into it and arrived at the set two hours late.

I asked if someone could find me something to eat, and one hundred assistants went running in all directions with no idea what to do. Three hours later, they still couldn't figure out how to find me food. Thousands of assistants came up to me to ask if I wanted anything but when I said 'food', they were too busy or important to do anything about it.

I was starving! Except for getting false eyelashes glued on me and receiving a full-face paint-over, nothing much was happening. So I googled where to find food and discovered there was a café twenty seconds away from where I was sitting. I went outside to get myself some breakfast.

Finally, at 2.00pm, I said my first line. 'Yummmm, I can hardly wait to hear the crunch!' As soon as I'd said it, more makeup was painted on me and millions of people started doing invisible things to the kitchen set in the empty ware-house. It could have been filmed in a real kitchen, but the producers liked spending as much money as they could (except for food for me), so they had built a complete kitchen unit – even though you only see me in front of a corner of the fridge.

I then repeated the line and the director shouted, 'Cut!' More makeup; more people rushing in and moving things around. A plate was moved a hairline to the left. Technicians started lighting another set.

This set was supposed to be an office (again, they could have filmed this in an actual office). The director shouted, 'Action' and I looked into the camera, saying with feeling, 'Can you hear the crunchy sound of the crunch?' I had to say that line 400 more times until it sounded like I was speaking Chinese.

My contract stipulated I had to stop shooting at exactly 4pm. This was so I could get to Ely Cathedral in time for the first night of my book tour. At around ten to four, I still had eight lines to say, so I just shouted them out as I threw myself into the car. Someone ran after me, recording every word.

Did I mention before that I'd be starting the book tour a mere thirty-six hours after returning from the retreat? No? Well, that's what I did. Not long after being back home I'm planning on ways to escape.

I live in a beautiful house. The problem is I can't stay there for long. For the last few years, I've been getting this sick sense of dread. I go to sleep, get up, and then I have to get out fast and go anywhere, even just to sit in a café. Put me in a hotel room, any hotel room, and I'm relaxed and a joy to be around.

When my kids were around, I could stay put. It was their home. I felt like I was finally in the park outside my childhood house playing baseball and bbq-ing. I was just like all the other mothers with kids. We were caught in clouds of love. Even when they become teens, you might roll your eyes and tear out your hair but you're still in those clouds of love. Then the kids go, and there's nothing left but having to face yourself with no clouds.

I was exhausted from jet lag. I asked the driver how long it was to Ely. He said that because of traffic, it would be three hours – if we were lucky. Okay, five hours later, still in the car, I had to go to the loo very badly. It was cold and black outside. We had passed absolutely no service station. I finally shouted for the driver to pull over, and to give me some paper. Any paper would do. Who would have thought that so soon after leaving the tranquillity of Spirit Rock, I would be clutching a piece of newspaper in a full King Lear-sized storm, and shitting on the side of the motorway?

I arrived late. The cathedral was full of people who had been waiting for hours to see me being interviewed. There was no changing room, so I changed clothes in front of a statue of Jesus looking miserable on his cross. And who could blame him?

I walked up to the altar to be interviewed by a kind but confused local priest about a book I couldn't even remember writing, let alone what it was about.

Do you know the size of Ely Cathedral? It's an entire continent of spires, 66 metres tall and 164 metres long. The cupola is actually in heaven. That's a lot of space to fill with your voice, especially when you haven't spoken for a month. There are four enormous wings in Ely Cathedral, like runways, jutting out in four directions. It would have been easy to look out at the audience if you could simultaneously talk and swivel your head 360 degrees, which you could do if your head was on a merry-go-round.

After the interview ended and I came down from the platform, I was confronted by a large group of very angry people. I thought they were complaining because there were no remaining copies to buy, but no, they were angry with me because the echo from my microphone had been blasting away and they hadn't been able to hear a word. My question is if they were sitting right in front of me and this wasn't a play, why didn't someone just stand up and say, 'Stop, I can't hear you'? I wanted to kill everyone, and this was in a cathedral! I couldn't even look the statue of Jesus in the face on the way out.

I was a wreck. I hadn't damaged myself by shooting the ad; what damaged me was starting a week-long book tour as soon as I finished shooting the ad. After the opening night disaster at Ely Cathedral, the nightmare continued.

I shouldn't have come back from the retreat and gone straight into the fast lane. I should have entered real life gently, not slap bang into a potato chip advert followed by a book tour. I know that now, it's called hindsight.

And to make the whole thing even more of a shitshow, I planned to go on a psilocybin mushroom trip seven days after returning from Spirit Rock. As soon as I heard you can't take mushrooms if you're on antidepressants (SSRIs) I went off my medication. (Big mistake.) I booked to go to Holland, which is the only place where it's legal to take those drugs. (There are more psilocybin retreats than people actually living there.)

I was no stranger to drugs. When I was eighteen I went to university. Free from my parents, except when they came to visit, or I had to go to Evanston for the holidays, I started to dabble in small amounts of LSD (LSD-LITE). I once dropped a small dose and I went to Disneyland with friends who were equally out of it. I remember we went on the ride 'Small Small World'. Now that's where you're on a small barge on a track moving down a canal, and on either side there are miniature automated dolls wearing their traditional costume representing almost every country in the world. It was a cacophony of weird accents. They were all singing 'Small Small World' in their own language.

But feeling invincible, I got off the barge to join the Hawaiian dolls in their hula dance. I was taken away by security, to be reprimanded and later released. It didn't stop there. At midnight, I watched Tinkerbell fly over the Magic Kingdom on a wire. I was so inspired, I insisted on finding whoever was in charge to apply for the job. When I found a manager, I aggressively told her that I'd like to apply for the role of Tinkerbell. She asked, 'Are you a professional aerialist?' I answered, 'Of course.' For some reason she didn't believe me and told me in a Disneyesque Minnie Mouse voice to get lost. I was devastated. My trip turned ugly when I saw Goofy and believed he was the Devil. I complained to the staff, who recognized me from the 'Small Small World' incident and Tinkerbell's replacement request and escorted me to the exit gates of Disneyland and threw me out.

About ten miles away from Disneyland, I jumped out of the car and ran into a field waving one of my left-over tickets over my head. When my friends tackled me to the ground (they had come down from the LSD, clearly I hadn't), I told them, 'It's okay, I know what I'm doing. I'm just going to use my spare tickets for my last ride.' They had to explain, 'It's a gasworks, Ruby, not another ride.'

I got home and after twelve hours of what they called 'lid flicks', I finally slept. Lid flicks are when you close your eyes after taking LSD and you get a light show of psychedelic, kaleidoscopic visuals on the back of your eyelids. At first thrilling, hours later you want to tear out your eyes.

These days, people are taking those same drugs for therapy. That would never have occurred to me while doing the hula in 'Small Small World'.

Clinic

23 May 2022

Shrink session
I really want to stop doing this EMDR.

S: *Tell me more about Ed. What does he give you?*

R: *Heat. I always felt like my family and I lived in the Antarctic and I spent my life freezing to death in the constant snow and ice. But Ed and his family had heat, and so I ran towards the flame. Ed came from a normal family. I found a home with them.*

S: *And you can't find that home now?*

R: *No. I don't know how to create it on my own. Ed's parents died and my kids have left.*

S: *We need to explore what home means to you.*

R: *Home was somewhere I needed to escape from, but the more I tried, the more I got caught. And the more I got caught, the harsher the punishment, and the harsher the punishment, the more I had to lie, and the more I had to lie, the more I was going to get caught.*

S: *Your whole trauma survival response is based on your perceived need to get away from home.*

R: *Yes. After my parents died, I sold the house to the next-door neighbours. It was razed to the ground. Bulldozers came and flattened it like brick roadkill. I went to visit there to make sure it was gone. It had no floor, just dirt with broken beer bottles spewed on it and garbage everywhere. My mother spent her life cleaning it and now it was just dirt, debris and bottles. It looked like houses after a bomb was dropped. Maybe this destroyed home was what my parents fled from during the war and that's what she pictured while she was on her hands and knees scrubbing perfectly clean floors. I'll never know. Now, whenever I see houses devastated by war on the news, I think that's where I lived. Ashes, rubbish and broken glass. There's home, yeah. When people tell me they can't wait to go home, it makes my skin crawl.*

S: *Okay. I think we're going to pause here and just allow some of this to process through. But think about what we're working on. We're working on this feeling that I need to get away but also that I don't know where to go. I think this is really interesting.*

*

Honestly, I wasn't sure I should go on a journey to trip on mushrooms at all. I find it particularly boring when people describe in detail their experiences on mushrooms. (They always mention a jaguar. Have you noticed that?) But so many people were claiming to have an 'awakening' from the experience, I thought, 'Come on, Ruby, get with it and show them how trendy you are, swallow a shroom.' Also, current research suggested that psilocybin could be a potential cure for depression. The paradox being that you can't take psilocybin if you're on antidepressants. So that's us depressives out.

I wanted a therapist to accompany me on this 'trip'. After I researched to find a Dutch therapist I liked, I booked flights to and from Holland. I was told the procedure would take five days. Day one they give you a mild dose to test your reaction. The following two days are for therapy to help consolidate the experience. On day four they give you the Herculean dose and day five is to rest.

The therapist insisted I do sessions with him by phone before I went to Rotterdam. Apparently this procedure is intended to make sure you're not going to go gaga on mushrooms. I agreed.

During the first session, when he asked about my childhood, I said I had loving and supportive parents who showered me with praise. When that wasn't enough information, I embroidered some details from American sitcoms. 'Mom makes cookies all the time, I can't stop her.' 'We sing carols around the Christmas tree. It's ever so jolly.' When the therapist asked me, 'Have you ever suffered from trauma?' I said, offended, 'Of course I don't have any trauma. I've been doing mindfulness for twenty years.' At the end of the session, he somehow believed I was trauma-free, which clearly I wasn't.

18 March 2022

I needed to pass a Covid test before flying. I did the test in the kitchen on the day of my departure. Guess who got a positive result? Me! I heard Ed say, 'This isn't good,' as we stood staring at those two lines that spell, 'You're screwed, you've got Covid.' I probably gave it to everyone who I signed a book for that past week. What can I say? To anyone who got an in-person signature on my book tour, I'm so sorry, I really thought it was a cold. Please God, don't strike me down.

Then Ed came back into the kitchen to tell me he also had tested positive for Covid. For the next ten days we were going to stay home, and you know my relationship with home, so I sat in the garden.

I had booked the next journey for a week after coming back from the now-cancelled mushroom trip, so I hoped we'd get over Covid fast. The trip was going to be swimming with whales.

Why would you think of swimming with whales, I hear you ask?

I'd found out about that particular adventure from a cameraman who works on Attenborough documentaries. I met him a few months earlier and asked him what was the most jaw-dropping experience he's ever had. He told me about his friend Captain Gene, who runs the only ship allowed into the area where you can swim with whales (otherwise they're protected from us dangerous humans). Without checking it out, I signed up with Captain Gene's Conscious Breath Adventures, with no idea what was in store. I only met the guy who gave me the tip once and he could have been joking or crazy, but for some reason I trusted him.

My happy place is when I'm about eighty feet under water. Whenever I've been scuba diving, I've begged to go down that far and then I refuse to ascend. I've had to have diving instructors drag me up because they say going that far below is dangerous. You get that warm sleepy feeling similar to an anaesthetic, which is my other happy place. The problem is you might not wake up, because at eighty feet if you stay too long, you fill up with nitrogen, which causes delirium and eventual poisoning. Oops! So here's why I chose this journey: I would be in the water, where I could dive deep and look a whale in the eye at the same time. What's not to love? And swimming with something weighing in at approximately thirty-five tons with an average length of thirty-nine metres might just humble me, show me how insignificant I am. If size mattered, this would teach me that I'd come in last.

24 March 2022

After a few days of lockdown, Ed broke the news that he had prostate cancer. He had never mentioned to me that the previous week he had gone in for a scan. They had just called him with the results. When Ed told me he had to have surgery and, even more worrying, he would have to take a test at the end of the week to find out if the cancer had spread, I didn't say much except I think I fainted standing up.

My world collapsed. I never thought about it but in that moment I realized I can't survive without Ed. (I've never told him; I hope he buys this book to find out.) I could try to be funny here by saying if he died, who would change the printer cartridge or the ceiling light bulbs? But I'll be straight with you, the only reason I've been able to live my life in free fall and why my kids are normal is because Ed can do it all. Ed is one of the only men I've ever trusted, and felt safe with. When I break down, he remains stoic. He doesn't crack under pressure. He comes from a military family and they know how to stay 'jolly brave and stiff upper lip it' even if they're about to be beheaded. They are what makes England great; that ability to have a cup of tea and a scone while doodlebug bombs are dropping all around. When I had depression twelve years ago, Ed took it on like a commando, which is what his father was. My kids have inherited this stoic feature – if they had more of my DNA, they would all be in cages by now, howling at the moon.

Sometimes I don't know why Ed sticks around. I shout instructions at him (not dissimilar to my mother). I'll bark, 'EEEEDDDD,' like an eagle squawking through a bullhorn, and then hand him things to fix or screw in. I don't know why he doesn't tell me to fuck off. I've aged and withered him. When we married, he was five years younger than me but from all the wear and tear of living with me, he now looks ten years older.

So now we had the threat of cancer and my mental illness bubbling away under the surface. We also had Covid. A triple header.

Clinic

25 May 2022

Shrink session

I'm doing another Zoom session with my shrink. I'm still not getting many clues as to who she is, but I will continue to investigate. She's back to her normal shirts again. I'm so glad. I feel I know her better in a shirt.

S: We haven't talked very much about when you were a teenager.

R: I know that I was plain, gawky and not popular. Boys mostly ignored me. If I had a crush on someone, I would start gabbling and not make sense – I was afraid they'd find out I was an idiot like my dad said I was. My dad was always telling me, 'You're a mess and so immature, Ruby.' I once stalked a guy who was in a rock band. I was completely obsessed. I'd call his house and I could hear him tell his friends, 'Tell her I'm not here.' It didn't stop me following him, I had no pride, even when he went out with his girlfriends. I finally followed him to Ohio on a visit to his family. I was supposed to be with my dad on holiday in Wisconsin for some 'us' time, like we didn't have enough of that. My dad got to Wisconsin first and kept calling my girlfriends to find out where I was. They told him I was on my way. When I finally got to Wisconsin a day later, he was waiting for me outside the hotel and in front of everyone, he did it again, he hammered into me in the middle of a road. It was like a show-down in a Western cowboy film but one of the cowboys was sixteen years old and didn't have a gun.

S: *What's the main picture of him waiting for you outside the hotel? What's the emotion it brings up?*

R: *Well, terror, terror. My heart is pounding. When I went towards him, he was shouting that I'm a liar. Then he just started clobbering me. He didn't think anything was wrong with it, he was always 'teaching me a lesson'. He'd say, 'If I don't discipline you, who will? This is for your own good.' He thought I had to be disciplined like our dog when he peed on the carpet. And then he'd say he was doing it out of love. You know, some people might think I have nothing to complain about. There were family vacations; my mother bought me nice clothes; I was taken to dance classes. On the one hand I had privilege. On the other I was treated like . . . I mean it was so shocking.*

★

Because of Ed's cancer diagnosis, it was now uncertain whether we would be going on the whale trip after all. Did

I mention, out of the kindness of my heart I had invited Ed to come on this journey? Well, I did. Friday, we would find out if Ed's cancer had spread. If the cancer had spread: no trip. If it hadn't, we could still go, and Ed would have his operation after we returned.

The evening before his appointment, I was hyperventilating. I was terrified Ed was going to die, but even so, I shouted at him because he ordered in the wrong food – I didn't want Chinese, I wanted Mexican – then the next morning, when we reached the doctor's office, Ed couldn't find a parking spot even though we'd passed six of them, and I shouted at him again. You'd think on the day he might get the worst news on earth, I'd give him a break?

I don't know what Ed was thinking. I would never have married me. When the oncologist was giving us the results of the test, Ed was his usual stoic self and I was blowing hard into a paper bag

But the news was good. The doctor told us Ed was clear. I was elated. So what did I do when we got back in the car? Did I say, 'Oh honey, I'm so happy for you. Why don't you just rest at home, and I'll take care of you?' No. I said, 'Ed, do you still want to go on the humpback trip? Or do you want me to go alone?' And Ed, God bless him, said, 'No, I'm coming with you.' So that night, we both packed our bags.

Once we arrived in the Dominican Republic, we were driven to a bizarre town called Puerto Plata. The builders had clearly given up, perhaps realizing that no one in their right mind would ever go there for a holiday. Puerto Plata was a seaside dump lined with half-built hotels and empty pools. There were open-air Mexican-style bars on every corner of the unpaved main street, filling the air with that eardrum-piercing sound of an announcer on the radio screaming about a special offer on hair gel. I think the locals do nothing for a living but put their feet on the table and chug beer. The women are nowhere in sight.

I was beginning to worry that Captain Gene's boat called *Sea Hunter* would turn out to be a lobster boat and we'd be sleeping in hammocks made of fish nets.

We met the first twelve guests on the dock. They were mostly good ol' Americans. One of the men, wearing an American flag for shorts, had a big ol' Texas personality, calling me 'honey' and everyone else 'y'all'. The other Americans, including a few elderly ladies who were travelling on their own, had big ol' personalities as well. I suspected they were all going to be highly entertaining and drunk most of the time.

When we finally boarded the *Sea Hunter*, I was relieved to find it was more like a yacht. A very big one. It had a living room, a small cinema, twelve classy wooden cabins with ensuite bathrooms and a white-tableclothed dining room.

Soon after we boarded, the remaining passengers walked in. I discovered they were a group of healers, and they had met on Facebook. Lena, a very svelte German, was the leader of the group. She wrote on Facebook that she was organizing a spiritual whale journey for a dozen people and these twelve healers had been the first to sign up. They were glamorous, and glowing. One of them was wearing a huge round ring made of crystals; thousands of tiny glittering shards of mirror on something the size of a tennis ball. I asked, 'Is that some sort of talisman?' She told me, 'It's for magic.' (Of course.)

Lena told me how she fell deeply in love with dolphins and whales on a trip to Hawaii: 'I was in the water up to my waist and suddenly hundreds of dolphins gathered around me and after a blinding flash, I found myself two miles out to sea without knowing how I got there.' Lena said that whales could download information from the universe because they remembered the beginning of evolution and had a much higher consciousness than humans. (Who doesn't?)

Silver Bank is a protected area about twenty-five by thirty-five square miles. The humpbacks come to Silver Bank to mate and after a year of pregnancy (ouch!) they swim back to Greenland, Norway or Iceland, wherever their journey began. They eat lots of herring there, and then they journey back to the Dominican Republic to mate again. Humpbacks can live to about 100 years so you can only imagine how many times they have to make this trip? I'm looking for meaning, they look for herring. There's a lesson in that but I don't know what it is.

THE *SEA HUNTER*
25 to 29 March 2022

Day 1

That night the ship set sail across the Atlantic, bound for the Silver Bank Sanctuary for whales. Ed and I and our fellow passengers would set anchor in the middle of the ocean for the next six days.

Looking back, I ask again how this man could have married me. I made him sleep on the upper bunk! May I just add here that Ed is three feet taller than me? This meant bumping his head on the ceiling whenever he sat up and having to climb up and down a ladder, while I just rolled in and out of bed.

Each day, two dive boats attached to the *Sea Hunter* would take us out to find some whales for us to swim with. The healers were on one dive boat and the Americans on the other. Ed and I were on the boat with America's finest. If any of us spotted a spurt, they'd shout to the rest, 'There's blow at twelve o'clock,' or 'There's a head at three o'clock,' and we'd all run like excited baboons. We'd shriek when a fifteen-foot dorsal was followed by a spurting geyser of water. Our jaws hit the ground at the sight of a hump the size of a dinosaur's back. To get a better view, we'd be hanging off the poles of the awnings. The sighting would end as the whale nose-dived back into the sea with a flick of its four-foot-wide tail.

When you spot a leviathan you see the iridescent blue under the water first. Then suddenly 150 tons of mammal propels out of the water, spins in the air like an obese ballet dancer, follows that move with a backward twist, and then, with a tsunami splash, returns to the sea.

When the whale gets close, you see tiny eyes on the sides of an enormous head, with bumps over the top the size of tennis balls. Nothing looks more alien than a humpback. When it wants to eat, its flat snout opens like an inflated accordion to swallow an entire population of herring, and then with a reverberating crunch, its mouth slams shut and the swallowed water gushes out of it like the Trevi Fountain.

My heart was soaring with happiness; it's what I wanted from this particular journey. Ed and I watched the spectacle like children, full of glee and awe. It's at such moments, I don't feel like a freak any more. I know that everyone around me is feeling exactly how I am: totally present and slightly vibrating with a feeling of aliveness.

Another thrilling whale showstopper is known as pec-slapping. That's when the whale lies on its back, sticks those gigantic pectorals in the air like jagged wings and slaps the water hard again and again, letting other males know, 'I am the biggest dick in this ocean, so back off.' If it's a female slapping the water she's flirting, saying, 'Come and get me boys, I'm feeling frisky.'

On the American boat, there was Darlene, a tough cookie, straight-talkin', hard-drinkin' gal who worked at an emergency call centre where she'd talk people through what to do if they encountered a dead body or how to help deliver a baby on the side of the motorway. When the waves were high, Darlene donned a black garbage bag. I was so inspired by her look that when the weather turned to torrential rain, I began to wear an off-the-shoulder garbage bag, too.

She described herself as 'pure filth' and suggested we get t-shirts made with whale-friendly expressions on them like 'Lookin' for blow' or 'Gimme head'. She had built her own house with her hands and lived there with her handicapped son. She had survived two violent husbands along with lung cancer. Though she'd had one of her lungs removed, Darlene dived fearlessly into the sea to swim with the whales and, even with a plastic tube in her nose for oxygen, she'd come out of the water heaving but happy.

Frank, the owner of the American flag shorts, was on our dive boat. He was so loud, I'm sure you could hear that drawl clear across Texas, where he hailed from. Frank was always in macho pose: legs apart, chest blown out, arms crossed, looking like Buzz Lightyear. Without giving pause, he streamed an endless monologue about how he once fought a grizzly bear, why he only ate four Brazil nuts a day, about his buddy who owned a gun ranch and, oh yeah, how Frank was arrested for selling coke and incarcerated. When his mother expressed her disappointment in him, he quit being a drug dealer the same day and took up a job in a deli. Shortly after that, he went into the extermination biz.

Frank and his best friend Rich ran the company together. I remember at Spirit Rock we had to swear an oath we'd never kill anything. Whenever we took a walk, we had to carry a special ant scooper-upper, just in case an ant crossed our path. Well, these boys provided us with 1,001 ways to kill anything and I mean anything. I asked Rich, 'What's the biggest pest you'd ever have to exterminate?' He came back with, 'My wife.' Darlene almost wet herself laughing.

There was also a handsome documentary maker named David on our boat. He looked like the Prince in every Disney film. Everyone on board (except Frank, because he's from Texas) wanted to have sex with him.

Cat – overly perky, smiley and blonde – was our dive master. Cat travelled from one international dive resort to the next. She appeared to be extremely comfortable with sharks – she thought Great Whites were 'cute' – and advised us that if we were confronted by a Great White, we should pet him on the nose to show we weren't afraid. She was also a free-diver who could hold her breath under water for over six minutes. Plus, she did a lot of pec-slapping during her time off.

One of Cat's jobs was to know the safest time to get into the water and approach the whales. The safest time was when they were taking a snooze. Cat knew how to spot a tired whale. Humpbacks can only swim for short distances because they use up so much energy, and when they get tired they sink to the bottom of the ocean for a rest. If the humpbacks don't rise up again after seventeen minutes, it means they have fallen into a deep sleep. We all sat on the dive boat like excited schoolgirls, counting the minutes and shouting 'Boo!' whenever the next humpback woke up and bobbed to the surface.

Finally, one of them stayed asleep. After seventeen minutes

had passed, Cat whispered (so as not to wake him up) for us to get our fins and snorkels on and get in the water quietly. Silently we descended. And there it was, as advertised, a sleeping whale. I swam up close. Then he woke up. As one of the largest mammals in the world glided up before my eyes, I said to myself, 'Remember this forever! You will never see anything like this again!' I had that breathtaking moment when the world stops and there is nothing – but nothing – going through your mind. You're in a heart-stopping state of pure joy.

I'm sure Ed thought a lot about his up-coming operation but, being a direct descendant of the 'stiff lip' brigade, he never spoke of it. Ed found Frank hilarious and loved hanging out with the Americans. They'd be chattering away about how well they all slept, their ailments and favourite Netflix box sets, while playing Monopoly for real money. (Frank usually cheated.)

Day 2

Since I could swing both ways, I'd sometimes leave the Americans and climb up a ladder to the upper deck to be with my other people, the healers. They spoke German, which is the language I spoke before I learned English. Every night the women sat in a circle, meditating to a recording of whale sounds. The whales start at the lowest bass note you've ever heard, then go to the highest squeak and go back down again and up again and on and on. Then the women would open their eyes and go around the circle one by one telling their deepest secrets. I could choose to be sarcastic but honestly it was incredibly touching to watch these women bonding on a deep level. Whoever spoke had everyone's undivided attention and there was love shining from everyone's eyes. Then they sang, making up the notes and harmonies as they went along. It sounded like a choir of mermaids calling to each other. Lena told the women to do 'a chain of love'. The idea is someone squeezes the hand of the person next to them and then that person squeezes the hand of whoever's next to them and so on, sending love around the circle.

One night when I climbed up the ladder to the upper deck, I saw to my surprise that the young documentary maker had been invited to join the healers' circle. One of the women was clutching David's hand and sobbing uncontrollably. She told us, in German, that she didn't trust men, while staring into David's eyes. He stared back with great compassion. This went on for an uncomfortably long time. Then, no longer weeping, she turned away to tell the group she could now trust at least one man. Then she asked Lena (luckily in German) if it was okay to ask David if she could lie on top of him? Everyone agreed that was a bad idea.

I climbed back down the ladder to rejoin the Americans. It was like going from yin to yang because I arrived just in time to hear Rich talking about the extermination company he owned with Frank. 'Whatever you've got besides your wife, I can eliminate it: cockroaches, bugs, ants and the worst, rats, mice, bats, snakes, pigeons who poop on cars. Alligators are my specialty. I lasso 'em by putting a wire around the gator's neck and then swing him into the back of my truck.'

He handed us cards that said: *Got a critter you want rid of? Call Rich.*

'If bats fly into a building, I sell my clients a big hoover to suck 'em back out into the night. For flies I sell 'em an air curtain so when the door opens, it just blows 'em out.'

These seemed expensive measures for a few intruders, but

who am I to judge? He described how to fumigate bugs and flies using gas pumps. I didn't ask what happened to the people with all that gas? He catered both for the rich and the poor. Local people, whom he lovingly calls 'trailer trash', 'come to me with crabs and pubic lice and, yup, I can even work with them and I give 'em free service'.

I had heard enough about clearing bats and bugs out of buildings with a gas pump, so I thought I'd head back to the healers. They wanted to manifest a 'singer' for the next day's whale watch. A whale is 'singing' when it hangs upside down in the water and emanates a sound that signals other whales.

I don't speak whale, so I couldn't tell you what the signal means. I assumed it was a mating call and whoever showed up and mounted you was your date for the evening. The healers disagreed with this interpretation. Lena told me, 'The singing is the way humpbacks download their ancient wisdom into whoever's listening, so they will find a purpose to their lives.' If a whale can do that, I clearly came to the right place. Lena told me, 'The whales know who you really are and give their wisdom to those they trust.' The healers then prayed to hear a singer the following day. I thought, if a whale can pass me some wisdom, I'm in.

Day 3

The next morning, instead of leaving with my usual crew, I joined the healers on their boat. They were waving frantically towards the sea to lure in any passing whales. Something must have worked, because some whales circled the boat and lifted up their giant pectorals. It was as if they were waving back at us. This didn't happen on the American boat.

Seeing the baby whales come closer to take a better look at us – and I mean, they were only three feet away – sent the women into a frenzy. They were dancing to house music like pagans possessed. We watched a tail flip-flop backwards and forwards for about an hour. It was as if a mermaid was head down under the waves, wagging her tail. We were told it was a mother telling her baby to get back to her because it had wandered too far away. Cat lowered a hydrophone into the water to listen in to the depths of the ocean, and there it was, loud and clear. Once they realized they had actually manifested a 'singer', the healers went bananas.

It wasn't a sweet whistling sound like I'd imagined. It began like a cow giving birth, and then the notes moved up to the tweet of a parakeet being strangled, and back down again, then up and down again. It sounded like, 'eeeeeee (high soprano note) aahhhhhhhh (descending note) ooooooooh (deep bass note)'.

I don't know if you've ever been on a small boat with women, wailing to find whales, but it was wild. This is what they had been manifesting since day one. Cat lowered the hydrophone and discovered we were directly above the singer. She said we could now put on our snorkels, fins and masks and she reminded us to jump in quietly. We did. And lo and behold there was the singer, with head down and tail up in the midst of creating that operatic lunatic cow/parakeet sound which vibrates through the water for miles. It also vibrates through you like you're just a human tuning fork. A concerto was coming out of an upside-down whale.

But we had to go. It was 6.30pm, and the sky was growing dark. Waves about five feet high were making the front of the boat rise almost straight up and then slam down. We had been hit by a squall. If we didn't leave the singing whale, we'd probably all drown. As the boat turned around, I hid under the covered part in the front, practically smashing my teeth with each slam. But it was worth losing my teeth because the experience was so out of this world.

Day 4

On our last night, Frank gave me four Brazil nuts and repeated his warning (he did this every night) that four were the right amount for selenium – which we need – but five would be lethal.

When I went to the upper deck, the women were sitting in a circle, taking turns to say goodbye to each other. One woman said she felt her soul was here, another said she always wanted to meet angels and now having got to know the other women, felt she had. Even though I'd divided my time between the Americans and the healers, I felt the same way. The Americans just chit-chatted, the women spoke from the heart, deep and honest. When it was my turn, I said, 'Being with all of you has been like being with twelve angels.' I was hugged profusely. When someone said, 'You are the thirteenth angel,' I felt honoured.

We held hands, and I'm sorry but I could feel the love pass through me this time and then I sent it on to my neighbour with a squeeze of a hand. One woman made the sound of a whale spewing water through its blowhole – 'phewwww' – and told us it was going to be her new attitude to life. It was the sound of letting go by this intense breathing out. We all started making the 'phewwww' sound of letting go in harmony.

Then one of the women came up the ladder and announced that someone in the crew had injured his back so badly that he couldn't move. He was incapacitated from the pain. If there was no improvement the following day, he would be asked to leave. She suggested they all go down and heal him. Carlos had a large family to feed. He couldn't afford to lose his job.

We all trooped down the ladder. The women asked Carlos, the injured crew member, if they could put their hands on him. He was embarrassed but he let them do it. The healers made a circle around him and placed their hands on his back. The rest of the male crew made a circle around the women. Then the women sang that strange mermaid song. A few of the crew broke down and wept.

Day 5

Usually I don't really go with the idea of healing with hands, but the following day I saw Carlos and he was standing tall, smiling and making that champion sign when you high-five the air. The Americans stopped their continuous chit-chat when I told them about the healing. Frank said it was mumbo-jumbo.

It was our last day together. A few hours after breakfast, I felt a searing pain shoot from my back tooth straight up into my gums. I'd had a bridge put in the week before we left on the trip, and something must have gone wrong. The agony was so unbearable that I asked the women if they'd mind putting their hands on me.

Twelve hands were placed on my head, arms, knees and back. It must have looked like one of those holy medieval paintings where angels in heaven are blessing baby Jesus. With the healers' hands on me, I could feel their warmth; I felt their protection. And I swear to you, the pain in my tooth faded.

Afterwards, one of them whispered to me, 'Thank mama.' I asked her to repeat what she said. She said it again, 'Thank your mama.' I was shocked, and I asked her, 'Why would you say that to me?' She told me, 'Your mother says she did the best she could.' The healer, it seems, was claiming to have insider knowledge of my parents. I wasn't sure if I wanted to hear any more.

In the old days, I would probably have taken notes and given them to Jennifer Saunders to stick into *Absolutely Fabulous*. I used to laugh at the idea of dead people giving out messages, but the healers had removed the pain of my toothache. It was a similar feeling when the schoolgirls protected me from my father. I loved the healers. I even loved the woman who claimed to be a reincarnation of a Mayan priestess.

The healer continued, 'You need to forgive all of the women in your family. They never intended their illness to pass to you.' This was unnerving: on my mother's side there was madness going all the way back through the ancestral line. She concluded with, 'Your mother and father want you to know that they love you. And they always have.'

This completely broke me. The Mayan priestess, who had been wearing the magic ring on the first day, squeezed my hand. Looking into my eyes, she whispered, 'You have a good soul.' Hers were the kind of eyes that pierce you to the heart. She continued, 'You are loved.' She took off her ring and placed it in my palm. I became very choked up, telling her that I couldn't accept her gift, but she insisted she wanted me to have it. At that moment I believed in everything.

Frank came over and gave the women four Brazil nuts each, which was quite an offering. The time had come for all of us to leave the *Sea Hunter*. The women formed a circle and had everyone join it, including the Americans and the entire crew. They led us in singing 'Amazing Grace', and then we all had to send love to the person beside us through our hands. I had

Frank next to me, and even though he was sometimes a pig, I sent him love. Then everyone – and I mean everyone – looked hard into each other's eyes like you don't do with strangers. The healers and the Americans were all of the same tribe. I watched as Ed, who has never been much for hugging, hugged each and every one of those healers. Then Captain Gene made a speech saying, 'I've never had such a weird passenger list but now it's become one of my favourite whale swimming cruises and I'll miss you all.'

So again, like Spirit Rock, at the end I felt that heat in my heart. I loved everyone, even Frank, who I'm sure is a Trumpster. I don't know if this sudden transformation came from swimming with whales or from being around healers. Maybe it was from both. We all promised to meet each other. I would come to Germany and Switzerland and stay with each one of them. I also signed up with Lena to go look for more whales in French Polynesia, where she was setting up a retreat. So far I've been in touch with no one. They loved me, I loved them back, what could go wrong?

P.S. Not everyone stayed out of touch. Frank is now emailing me regularly, calling me 'sweet pea' and reminding me about the four Brazil nuts.

My downfall was that I booked all my journeys too close to one another, sometimes only a few days apart. There was no time for the experience to seep in. Who in their right mind does something like that? When I tell my fellow inmates in the clinic, even they say it's crazy, which is high praise indeed.

Clinic

26 May 2022

Shrink session

The shrink is wearing a summer dress today. It's light blue. It has an open collar and buttons down the front. I didn't think she'd be a summer dress sort of person but then what do I know? I was tempted to ask about her choice of clothing but a little voice in my head told me to not go there.

R: *Who goes from one journey to the next at the speed of light? Me. Why is that?*

S: *I think you go to these endless places always thinking, 'Is that where I belong?' 'Is this where I belong?' You're looking outside of yourself for something that's an internal problem. At the heart of this is how we help you to find home within yourself.*

R: *I think it was subconsciously instilled in me at an early age that I had better find some place of safety in the outside world.*

S: *Your childhood experience is 'I'm on my own in this haunted house that I'm meant to call home and I need to escape. But if I get out, I've got no means of looking after myself, and they're going to come after me.' You're compelled to re-enact the same process over and over: 'I can't settle; I can't feel at home so I need to get out; I need to plan something.' As soon as you start planning something, you start to feel better. But you won't find a geographical solution to what is a psychological problem. That's the work that we need to do.*

*

After my parents died, I ravaged the house, stuffed their history into garbage bags and burnt it all. The last thing I did was to carry a round heavy clock that hung by a chain from our living-room ceiling. The clock was the weight of a plane. Ed filmed me as I twirled it over my head like a cowboy roping in cattle and let it fly into the lake. I threw it into the lake, thinking that's the end of my childhood, without thinking I would carry my childhood with me.

I hate digging up all the horror shows from my past but the shrink says the only way to deal with depression is to face the music, because if the memories remain buried in my unconscious, it will be like living with a timebomb, that one day when I least expect it, will detonate.

27 May 2022

At art therapy, we go around the circle, as we do at the start of every class, to check in how we feel. It's almost like the 'chain of love'. Most of us feel like shit.

Then we're told we have forty-five minutes to express ourselves on paper. I can't draw anything, only stick figures that could have been done by a child of four with a learning disability. I can, however, channel Picasso. I've done it several times before. I go online to find one of his paintings and after swirling the oils and imitating the features, I've created an exact – and I mean, you can't tell the difference – an exact replica of a Picasso.

After an hour we're told to stop. I think my fellow inmates are going to faint when they see what I've created. It doesn't happen. They hold up what they've painted, and I shrivel. Every single person in the art class has painted something so deep and meaningful, I'm suddenly ashamed of my skills at counterfeiting.

This is the good news about people touched by madness. Give them an easel and a brush and genius happens. One girl painted a finely detailed cherry blossom tree in Japanese style: it was growing in on itself, like it was eating itself alive. A guy who always looked so sad and withdrawn drew an elephant chained to his heart so you couldn't tell who was dragging whom.

Others drew intricate helixes, mandalas and images created out of the minds of the deepest of souls. I held up my Picasso and when asked what it represented, I could only say, 'It represents nothing.' I was showing off my skills in imitation. Everyone was an artist and I was a counterfeiter, a fraudster. I went to my ward and took another tranquillizer.

4

Refugees

*We need to let go of the life we have planned to live the one that is
waiting for us.*

– Joseph Campbell

I left my humpback sisters telling me how beautiful my soul
was – they said it in German so I may not have it completely
right – and I was clutching my magic ring, when Ed and I
boarded the plane for our return flight to the UK. I spent the
next few hours wrapped in the same cocoon of peace and
love I'd been in when I left Spirit Rock the month before. The
happiness lasted until the plane landed.

It wasn't my fault for losing it this time. I was in agony.
The shooting pains coming from the place where I'd had my
dental work the week before were so terrible that I started
confessing to war crimes. Compassion for the human race
had been replaced by rage towards the dentist who had
screwed up and charged me a fortune.

'I don't care how many heads, crowns or orthodontic procedures have to roll,' I barked at his secretary. 'This is an
emergency!' They got me into surgery that afternoon. When
I woke, I was in bliss again but only because of the co-
codamol. I had gone from a 'beautiful soul' to a drug addict

in two days. (Co-codamol is one of the heaviest painkillers outside of Oxycontin.)

I went back to my old routine, filling in any cracks of my day to make sure there was no airtime. The nonsensical 'to do' list was gaining momentum. I had no time to reflect on what I had learned on my journeys. I was a swirling dervish of chores that had to be done immediately: buy a selfie stick (would never use), get sports socks (why?), make an appointment for pottery class (never went), make reservations at various Airbnbs around the world (no plans for going to any of them). I had gone past my tipping point. Too busy to notice something was 'rotten in the state of Denmark'. Hamlet had depression too, so he should know.

Clinic

28 May 2022

Shrink session

The shrink is wearing the weirdest silk shirt. It's got a white background with things that look like small sausages tied up in red rope all over it. (Freud would have a field day with this one.) She asks me if I can remember my mother picking me up when I was a baby. And I realized I can't. Don't feel sorry for me (well, do if you want and have time), but I think she was pretty pissed off that I ruined her model-like shape. She said she wore her belt at the tightest notch, even when she was pregnant.

R: Why is it so important to be picked up by the mother or caregiver or whoever?

S: *If the baby isn't held, made eye contact with or spoken to softly, the baby won't know how to self-soothe when she becomes an adult.*

R: *I don't know what you mean by self-soothe? Is it like taking a bubble bath with candles? Okay, sorry, I know what you mean, I just can't do it to myself. Is that why I feel better when I'm surrounded by women? They can soothe for me?*

S: *I would say that's the case. Was there anyone at home who nurtured you?*

R: *Omi, which means grandmother in German, she was my saviour. I loved her. Omi was cute and all roly-poly and full of love for me in that sweet grandma kind of way. She did what she could to protect me. One time she walked in when my mother was hitting me and I can remember her trying to pry my mother's hands off me, shouting that she must not beat her child.*

S: *Anyone else?*

R: *Starting when I was about ten, I'd sneak over to my Aunt Harriet's house. Harriet Hambourger. Isn't that weird, my dad was in the sausage business and all my relatives were hambourgers? Spelt differently, but still weird. She was one of my saviours.*

Harriet lived in a simple suburban house; nothing fancy but it felt like a real home. I remember her fridge was stuffed with food, whereas there was hardly anything inside our fridge except Cuban cigars and a jar of mayonnaise with a sell-by date of 1952. Aunt Harriet was in her seventies, which seemed very old to me, but she had a glow about her. She knew how crazy my parents were. She'd ask me questions. She'd listen. I felt heard.

After I'd been at her house a few minutes, right on cue, my dad would drive up. He'd have figured out I'd gone to Aunt Harriet's, and he would drag me back to our house. My mother hated that I went to Harriet's. She'd say, 'Why did you go there of all places? What's so special about Harriet? She has no chic. She's a nobody.' May I remind you, it was our relatives in America, the Hambourgers, who got my mother, father and grandmother out of Vienna.

My mother was very 'chic'. She bought me clothes she thought would make me look cute, like she was dressing up a doll. She was disappointed that I wasn't beautiful and didn't have a model-like figure. As far as my father was concerned I was some ugly duckling, he was always telling me what a 'sad sack' I was.

29 May 2022

Tonight we are going to eat Chinese with Ed. My daughters hold my hand as we walk. I ask the girls about how their rehearsals are going for the Edinburgh Festival in a few months. Their act is called 'Siblings', very 'French and Saunders' but more bizarre.

I'm proud of them, but when I watch them perform I'm a nervous wreck. Someone took a video of me once from the back of the stage. My face was contorted in terror, hands over my mouth to stop the screams. I look like that because I know how painful it is to fail, when there's silence during a show and your insides drop out while you're performing . . . Then when you succeed, you feel love pouring at you from the audience for making them laugh. This is why you do something that at times is sick-making.

I'm always trying to give the girls suggestions but they refuse all notes because I know nothing. They aren't as desperate as I was to make it. They're just happy and have a great time performing. I thank Ed's genes for breaking generations of madness in my family.

In the restaurant when I laugh at their jokes, it sounds hollow, even to my ear. I'm trying to act like I used to be before the depression, but we all know that mommy is missing and someone else has possessed her. They keep asking when I'm coming home. I'm the last person to know that.

On that last day aboard the boat, the healer had told me my mother said she did all she could. Those words kept echoing inside my head. This conversation was haunting me. She'd told me my mother loved me. Had I been too hard on her?

I imagined her as the girl I'd seen in photos: long golden hair, azure blue eyes and porcelain skin. In the photos she made Greta Garbo look like a floor-mop.

She was incredibly popular at school; if they'd had such a thing in her day, she would have been Prom Queen. If we were in the same class, she would have ignored me. My mother was brilliant, got straight A's, spoke eight languages and knew Goethe by heart. I was in the 'slower, remedial duh' group at school. No one read in the 'duh' class so we just had to hold up our favourite pictures.

She was so beautiful – and Aryan-looking – that when she was on the train (the papers for America presumably safely tucked away in her handbag) an entire row of Nazis stood up so she could lie down to sleep.

People who knew her back then told me that she was the 'it' girl of Vienna. I've seen photos of her skiing in St Moritz with a dashing Italian soldier's arm around her; on the Riviera sailing with a General; in Salzburg at the Opera with a soldier who looked a lot like Mussolini. All those handsome men stood tall, and their backs were iron-rod straight, square-jawed with vicious charm. She obviously liked a man in a uniform.

Imagine having to leave all that behind, to suddenly have to pack your bags and flee. Flee fast! I think that urge to flee is embedded in my DNA. I can clean out my closet, get rid of any sign that I lived there, and be out the door in less than six minutes. When I'm going somewhere, I like to start packing when the taxi pulls up to get a few hits of that delicious adrenaline rush. Sometimes, I even throw in a shower before I start packing when the taxi arrives and starts the wild honking. I'm sure this is a leftover trait from my relatives in the old country having to not just pack clothes, but tie their furniture and pianos on their backs and scram.

My father was very clever in how he survived the war. There were times his name would appear on the list of those who were to be sent to a camp. He never was taken away because whenever the Gestapo showed up to read the names from the latest 'who's being taken away' list, he'd fall over and pretend to have an epileptic fit. The soldiers couldn't be bothered to lift and carry a convulsing man so they left him convulsing away until the next time.

My parents never talked to me about their experiences during the war, but even though they didn't say anything specific, I could taste their fear. I didn't need to see any films about the Holocaust (and never have), the images living in my mind are enough. I have *Schindler's List* on a loop tape playing in my head.

It's ironic that my parents ran from Europe to escape the war and I ran to Europe to escape them.

31 May 2022

My son Max comes. He's scared that I'm sick but he pretends it's perfectly normal to visit your mother on a mental ward. He's done a search and found an eccentric coffee shop he thinks I'd like. He knows I love the unusual and kitsch and last week he found it. It's decorated like I've crashed a sixteen-year-old's birthday party, with balloons, streamers, tinsel, blinking coloured lights, and everywhere you look, cakes in the shapes of cartoon characters. Max knows how to cheer me up.

1 June 2022

Shrink session

R: *Yesterday I took a short walk on my own. I passed a hotel, with a restaurant out front. There was a group of women sitting around a table. They were drinking champagne. They were all dressed up, and they were laughing. It looked like they were having such a good time, and I felt like joining in. Then I wondered what they'd think of me if I joined them. Would they think I'm too weird? That I didn't belong? Would I have a clue what they're talking about?*

S: *Okay. So just connect into that feeling. What's the energy around that feeling of 'I can't fit in. I don't fit in.'*

R: *Well, extreme loneliness. I don't know where I belong.*

S: *Okay. So part of what you're trying to get away from is extreme loneliness. And then the other part is envy. What are you envying?*

R: *I wish my life looked more like theirs. What's coming up is I'm feeling that because of how my parents were, I'm envious of others.*

S: *Okay, take that image of the friends in the café laughing, and the tension you felt between wanting to join in, and believing they would reject you. What comes into your mind?*

R: *That I'm a freak and they'll catch me out. Envy and anger that I don't fit in. I don't even know what conversation to have.*

S: *Okay, so hold this image of the café where people are having fun, and now connect it to your fear they'll find out you're a freak. We're going to use that as a portal into your trauma.*

★

2 June 2022

I went to morning yoga class, which they offer here to unfold us from being bedridden. Most of us just stand there with our legs apart. We're fighting gravity and that's all that matters. If you can stand up and walk, you've reached the next level.

During one of the classes, I notice a girl next to me wearing a short-sleeved shirt so I can see her arms are cut to shreds. I take her upstairs. She's incredibly beautiful and tells me she comes from Mumbai. She tells me some horror stories of her experiences on the ward. I call in a nurse to take notes. I'm going to have to report this because the girl is too afraid to do it herself.

While we're talking, I notice another girl in the kitchen.

Wherever I go, there she is. And suddenly out of nowhere, she says, 'Oh, my God, I've just googled you and I know who you are. I can't believe it.'

In my arrogance, obviously I think she's talking about me, but no, she's focused on the cut-up girl. She says – coming out of her shell fast – 'You're one of the most famous singers in India. I watch you on Asian BBC. My dream is to become a famous singer, could I sing for you?' And the girl, who's in shock anyway, says, 'When?' And the other girl says, 'Now.' So off they go to a communal room.

The nurse and I don't know what to say. I follow her and open the door a little; I see the back of the Indian girl's head and standing before her is the snail singing in a low strangled hum like a drain that's been clogged and just opened after ten years. I feel terrible I caused this.

Later I googled the girl and, yes, she is one of the most famous singers in India, which means she has over a billion hits. That puts me in my place, thinking the fan recognized me from my television days. I'm such an asshole.

My father's escape from Vienna took longer and was more difficult than my mother's. He tried to get entry to Australia, the UK, Africa and was unanimously turned down. He tried to ski into Switzerland (which was neutral) from Austria, but 16,000 other Jews had the same idea, and he was promptly picked up and arrested. He escaped from prison and eventually got to Belgium, where he stowed away on an ocean liner going to the New York World's Fair. He must have been petrified of being caught on that ship, he had no papers, and if he had been found stowing away, he would never have been allowed into the USA or would have been U-turned back to the old country and shot.

Once he was reunited with my mother in Chicago, my

aunt in Vienna begged them to help her family get to the United States. I'd always assumed the reason my parents never mentioned that was because they couldn't be of any help. But during the filming of *Who Do You Think You Are?* (a television show where they revealed my genealogy to me by taking me to Vienna), I learned how hard my parents tried to save her. They sent my aunt and her family the correct papers but by the time the documents arrived, the Nazis had closed the borders. No one could leave the country because it was too late, and the family was exterminated. I learned one member of the family was a boy called Max. My parents had never mentioned him to me, even though coincidentally I named my son Max.

During the filming, they took me to the synagogue where my parents got married. This was on Kristallnacht, the night the ghetto was bombed. My parents never mentioned it. I grew up assuming Kristallnacht was the night the Jews brought out all their crystal and went from door to door showing it to each other and then dropped it.

Did my parents love each other? I guess they did once before it got ugly. They brought the war into our kitchen, where they'd have screaming matches. I was piggy in the middle. My mother would say, 'I don't know what's wrong with her? Maybe from the bomb. Her head is not on right. And those teeth? She looks like a squirrel.'

My dad would throw in, 'Who's going to marry her when her behind is as big as a house?'

My mother then clanged in with, 'Why do you have to eat so much, Ruby?'

Dad: *That's why her behind is as big as a bus. It's an abomination.*

Mom: *I had a beautiful figure when I was in Vienna. Do you remember, Eddie? (My dad's name.)*

Dad: *That's why I married you, Berta, you were beautiful but always crazy. That's how you'll end up, Ruby, crazy like your mother.*

*

They were both demented. In those days no one knew much about madness. I don't know if my parents became mentally disturbed from being refugees, or if they were always that way.

It's probably not that surprising given my home life, but ever since I was young, I've always been fascinated by mental illness. I stole a book from my grade school library called *This is Mental Illness*. It's about fifty-five years overdue. I must owe them millions. (Hopefully, the librarian from Evanston Junior High isn't reading this book and won't start hunting me down.) So when I found out that I came from a long line of mentally ill relatives, I wasn't that surprised.

When she was old and in a nursing home, I took my mother to see a psychiatrist because she was writing 10,000-dollar cheques to the window cleaner and accidentally setting fire to the curtains. He prescribed Prozac and her nurse began sprinkling it in her food. From then on, my mother became the most popular girl in the nursing home. Everyone loved her. I couldn't help thinking that if Prozac had been around sixty years earlier, I wouldn't have been so screwed up.

3 June 2022

I walked to the hotel next door. They know me there as the crazy person in pyjamas. Even though I'm wearing a coat, somehow they can still tell I'm in pyjamas.

I started yelling at a waitress for not letting me order salad. She said they don't serve it. I said I have it here most days. Two Nigerians said they came in every day, too, and they had salad. They were on my side. We bonded over the salad.

The three of us reported the waitress to the maître d', saying her attitude was appalling.

The salad arrived. I didn't pay for mine because of the way I was treated. I found out later they had to pay for me. They probably think I do that every day.

I wonder if the Nigerians were also from the clinic.

4 June 2022

Shrink session

The shrink looks the same as always. I wonder sometimes if she ever leaves her chair.

R: *My father used to tell me I would go insane. He said I would go insane because I have a mind like my mother's.*

S: *He told you you'd be insane?*

R: *He said by fifty I'd be insane. So he's off by twenty years. That's why he wasn't going to leave me an inheritance. He didn't want to leave me any money because he knew that I'd be crazy.*

S: *What kind of parent says that to their kid?*

R: *I don't know what he was trying to do. Except he would have liked me to go insane and he got it. He'd laugh and roll his eyes: 'Ruby wants to be an actress. Look at her!' He told people he only sent me to drama school because it cost less than having me committed to a mental institution.*

We were interrupted when the shrink's dog (a black Labrador) jumped into the screen and on to her lap. She lovingly tells him that this is no place for dogs and she'll walk him later. I'm confused how she's going to do that, since I don't think of her with a lower half.

R: *My parents sent me to a shrink at age fourteen. They wanted to 'normalize' me.*

S: *Normalize you? They should have celebrated your uniqueness.*

R: *They wanted me to keep up with everyone else, and be more like the popular girls at school. But when I met Dr Levy, the first words he said to me as I walked into his office were, 'Your mother is a basket case.'*

⋆

5 June 2022

Today I'm going for another transcranial experience. After my first one, I was told that one of the side-effects was tiredness. I told them I don't have any side-effects. An hour later I was face down in a plateful of lasagne.

Ed comes to deliver other items from the list, which includes my bike. He has to carry it up four flights of stairs, as the elevator still hasn't been repaired. I realize he didn't bring the brownies I ordered and he apologizes profusely, promising to return with the said brownies. I think when I'm mentally ill, he tries to acquiesce to all my whims in case I try to stab him.

6 June 2022

Shrink session

Today the shrink is sitting in a different room with light Ikea-type shelves behind her. I asked her where she was. She said she was in one of her kids' rooms because the windows in her office had to be replaced. Did she break them? Did some patient throw a stone through them? (I was lost in a fantasy about what happened to those windows?)

S: *It must have been very confusing for a little girl. Your mother waking you up at night crying and telling you she loves you, and then –*

R: *– yes, then yelling because I didn't fold things correctly. And just tearing out all the clothes from my drawers. Tearing them out and then refolding them. Omi knew something was wrong with my mother. When I was little, she'd let me crawl into bed with her. But my dad wouldn't let me sleep there so he'd yank me out of bed by my legs. Eventually he injured his back from pulling me out so often. He had back problems for the rest of his life, which I was glad about.*

S: *I want you to follow the ball with your eyes back and forth on the screen. Imagine meeting your eight-year-old self. She's sitting on her bed. Will you sit beside her? We know that she's frightened. Could you reassure her that you're able to protect her?*

R: No. I'd be lying because other people are going to damage her later.

S: Isn't there a part of you that wants to protect her like you did with your own children?

R: No. There is part of me that wants to kick her for being so weak. What do you want me to do? Pick her up and give her a big hug and then we both start crying? If this was a film, I'd walk out right about now. You're setting me up.

S: Just be with her. Ask her what she wants.

R: Why?

S: This little girl is the one who needs you to be arranging events and making her look successful. It's coming from her. You're driven to get the approval of all these different people because she needs to feel okay. She has a lot of power over you.

R: So I'm like her PA? I'm going to be stuck with organizing her life forever?

S: I'm saying that a lot of what you're doing is to soothe her.

R: She keeps me too busy.

S: It's had a really negative impact on your everyday life. You end up being driven, making arrangements with people you don't want to spend time with simply to keep her soothed.

R: She's draining my energy.

S: Right now, you're a slave to her needs. She is very dominant in your system. You get confused as to why you keep making all these plans with so many people? You're doing it all for her. And she can't step down unless a wiser part of you steps up to say, 'Look,

I understand. But I'm not going to phone anyone just because you're afraid of being alone.'

R: *That's why I constantly want to leave all the time. If I've left town, the eight-year-old can't get her own way.*

★

Is it a coincidence, or are there any coincidences, that the healers mentioned my parents and the journey looking for meaning that I had arranged after the whales was to work with refugees? I felt a compulsion to work with refugees because my parents escaped to America from Austria. It was only because of kind relatives that they got out, which is lucky because otherwise I wouldn't be writing this book – or be in existance. I felt I should help the inmates the way those relatives helped my parents, and also have a chance to use my compassion muscle for a change. Maybe I went there for selfish reasons but those refugees don't care why you're there; the fact is you're there. I got deeply involved with some of them. I listened to their stories and eventually I tried to help a family get their relatives out of Afghanistan. Read on to see what happened.

Another reason I decided to work with refugees is that I was sick of people yapping with each other at dinner parties about the refugee crisis. I've always thought, 'If it really bothers you, get off your ass and do something! Don't just throw quotes at me from the same newspaper I read this morning.' I didn't want to see them in all their misery on the BBC News any more. I wanted to listen to their stories first hand. How they escaped from Iran, Somalia, Syria or Afghanistan and made it to Greece in a lifeboat. I wanted to feel a human connection, and not just glimpse refugees as a piece of film footage.

Three years ago I went to a refugee camp in Samos. When I was there, I had the privilege of working beside nurses, teachers and heads of charities who worked with such compassion it took your breath away. When you're near people doing that, you catch being compassionate, like it's a virus. A good one. I wanted to experience that again; being near the most generous people on earth who don't expect reward or approval; they simply want to be kind.

I decided I'd return to Greece to volunteer at another refugee camp. Maybe it was a selfish act to make myself feel better, but refugees aren't going to ask you your motive, they're happy you cared enough to show up.

It had been relatively easy to volunteer for my last trip to Samos, but this time I was told that the Greek government wasn't allowing in any more volunteers. It was partly because they didn't want anyone to report on the atrocious conditions in the camps. Another reason for the 'no volunteers' policy was that some volunteers were doing more harm than good. They were trying to convert the refugees to their religious beliefs, or bringing in food without a plan on how to distribute it (which caused mayhem). Riots had broken out when there wasn't enough food to go around.

Another problem was the number of female volunteers who wanted to have relationships with male refugees. Some of the men proposed marriage and the girls accepted. There wasn't a happily ever after ending. (Surprise, surprise.) After the girls brought them back home having arranged their passports, their 'fiancés' ditched them at the altar.

So, there would be no more volunteers, only doctors or

NGOs. But on my last trip I had met someone, who knew someone else, whose cousin knew someone – the chain went further and further up to the well-connected – and he gave me the number of D, a woman who worked in cahoots with the Greek officials.

She was the consummate underground fixer, getting supplies for the camps from anywhere in Europe with the snap of her fingers. The Greek government had turned a blind eye to her activities for thirty years because she accomplished what they couldn't – providing basics for the refugees.

If women were permitted in the Mafia, D would have been one. Her networks brought in truckloads of nappies, baby food, sanitary towels, school books, clothes, blankets, etc.

She was known as the 'soul of the camp'. It's all about knowing someone, who knows someone, who's cousins with someone. I scored with D, who invited me, because she could spot I too was a bulldozer, over the phone, to be her assistant at the refugee camp where she ruled.

Refugee camp

The camp was forty miles outside of Athens. I rented a car at the airport and followed road signs written in hieroglyphics. I exited at almost every ramp in fear of heading the wrong way, barking to anyone passing in English, 'Where am I?' They laughed at the idiot speaking something incomprehensible. D had given me the name of a hotel close to the camp. After many hours of pleading out the window of the car waving maps, I miraculously found it. I don't know if you've seen *The Shining*, but that was the vibe. Weird David Lynch music filled the air.

No furniture. Endless empty shiny floors leading to an

empty bar and an empty outdoor swimming pool. At one end of a hall going nowhere, there was a giant made of red velvet. His head was held up by a thin pole two feet above his neck. I nearly fainted. (I found out later it was an art installation.) I eventually located a human in the lobby. His head was connected, unlike his eyes, which were going all whirly-burly in all directions but one – to my face.

My room was normal except for the shower, which had more than twelve nozzles. Stepping into it, I felt like I was going into a car wash where my organs could be whooshed out of my body.

The next day I drove through majestic mountains and enchanting, sheep-clad villages. Various versions of Zorba were drinking at outdoor bars. I finally got to the camp, which was surrounded by barbed wire. A guard stood at the entrance, keeping everyone who wasn't a refugee out. D was there to meet me and with a flick of her finger, the gates flew open to let me in.

There is that moment when you enter and you could be back in time, in some ancient Bedouin slum in the desert. There were large circus-like tents separated by a few shacks made of rusted corrugated tin. The beating sun had turned the ground into hard dust. I tried to smile at the people passing me, instead of just gaping at them. Those who caught my eye smiled back.

I went into a circus tent and found myself in a maze of dirty hanging sheets. Those unlucky enough not to live in one of the tin cans could live in the big tent with four sheets as walls. Each family, no matter how many members there were, got one room the size of a closet. Inside the tent, 200 families huddled within those squares of bedsheets.

In winter they freeze and in summer they fry. They cooked on a primitive iron age stove and slept on a blanket on the dirt floor where rats scampered. If there was an outbreak of a disease, it would take seconds to infect everyone. As there were no walls, there was no privacy. If someone spoke, you heard every word, sound, sob, cough. No one seemed to move around much during the day. When I'd peek into the sheeted squares, the men and women would immediately invite me in for tea. They have nothing and yet they invite you for tea. I always accepted. I made friends with a woman who invited me to her home/sheet cubicle. The mattress on the floor was covered with toys and dolls. She explained in broken English and mime that her husband and baby daughter were caught crossing a border and taken to some internment camp in Turkey. She had no idea where and probably never will, as they've lost all connection. The toys on the bed were to remind her of the life she'll never have, and the family she'll never find. She showed me photos of her lost family but instead of breaking down, she served me her last cookie on a doily, on a plate with a napkin.

The first few days I helped D in the 'boutique', which was a couple of tables piled high with used unwashed clothes. I had just separated the baby, toddler and teenager clothes, and was trying to fold them neatly when the doors opened and a horde just ran in and grabbed as much as they could. I was about to tell them off for making a mess out of my neat piles when a lightbulb went on in my head. The refugees had nothing. Whatever they'd once owned had been taken away, so now they were doing the grabbing and in their circumstances, I would have grabbed too.

I recorded conversations I had with some of the refugees on my iPhone. They didn't hold back; everyone wanted to tell their story because they could see I cared enough to listen and God, did I care. When someone trusts me enough to open their heart, I have to open mine. Their circumstances were as far away from mine as it gets, but I felt a closeness. I kept thinking what if the Americans had shut the gates on my parents, telling them, 'Good luck with the Nazis'?

D told me to stop folding clothes, she wanted me to keep talking to the refugees. She could see that we connected.

Conversation 1

I'm with a teenager who worked in the boutique with me on my first day. I'll call him F.

R: *How long have you been here?*

F: *Just seven or eight months ago we come here from Turkey to Greece. I'm from Afghanistan. From Kabul City.*

R: *How did you get here? Do you mind me asking?*

F: *Walking. For six days it was really hard but right now we are here, and I feel safe.*

R: *Did you come with your family?*

F: *No, my father sent me and my big brother here because my father don't have more money to come with all of our family. Then he choose to send me and my brother.*

R: *Do you feel like you're in shock a little bit?*

F: *Exactly, yeah. Like ten or eleven days ago was my birthday. I just become seventeen years old. But in this age, I saw a lot of things that I wish I did not and this is a little bit hard. Yeah, a* sixteen-year-old shouldn't see that. I don't know anything about governments. But Taliban, I think they are not human. Two times when I was in Kabul City, two times I see bomb go off with my eyes. And I shouldn't have seen what I seen. I see broken people, arms, heads . . .

R: *So you walked here? Did you use Google maps?*

F: *Yes, exactly, and we use GPS. So yeah, we was walking for six days, nothing, just jungle. Sleep on the ground. Our water was really low. When I was walking, I was just thinking about my goals. And that was making me strong. I will bring my family. Also one of my important goals in my life is football. I will play football and I will make money and I will be saved.*

R: *How would you make money by playing football?*

F: *No, not right now. But in the future. I will make my body good and they will pay me and I will be a football star. This is for sure.*

*

Conversation 2

I'm now talking to L, who's in his twenties. They all speak numerous languages.

R: *How did you get here?*

L: *I lived in Lesbos island and I came there and was stuck in the middle of the sea. I call to the police because in that boat, only I can speak English. I tell them we have got two pregnant women. Then one of them, the water break. I call to the police. I said to them, we got this problem. If it's possible, don't help us, only help that woman and the baby. They said wait and gave the phone to someone who says he's a doctor.*

R: *So she's in labour?*

L: *He says you can born baby in middle of the sea. And I don't tell them I'm qualified doctor. He says, 'Are you feeling head of baby?' I lie to them and said, 'No. The baby twisted and I feel the feet,' so that they think it's an emergency and come to help us. When they come the police say to us, 'The reasons for helping is that woman and the baby. But after we take her off, you all will go back to Turkey.' Now we are in Lesvos and I am only persons between 158 persons who can speak English. They ask if I was the one who call them and I say 'yes'. After that they put me in jail without any reasons. Five months and twenty-two days without any sunlight.*

R: *With no explanation?*

L: *Nothing. I tried five times to kill myself. I close my lips. I stopped eating and drinking for a long time. And after that they brought me to the interview room. I'm now under the torture. All week for six months. They do that and they broke my legs in twenty days, three times. They tried to find out if I said bad things but I said you must prove I did this.*

R: *What did they say you did?*

L: *That I talk against my government and they say I have secret data. I said have you proof that I have it and after torture they can't find out anything and they released me. Three of my friends were also arrested in Greece and they deported them back to Iran and they executed. And I'm scared about that because when I arrested, Iranian government called to my family and they said* *you can see your son as soon as possible but he will be a dead body.*

★

Conversation 3

I spoke to a little girl wearing a hijab and Western clothes.

R: *You're twelve?*

C: *Yes, I'm twelve.*

R: *Oh my God. I thought you were much older.*

C: *Oh, really? I think that's bad because I should look like my age.*

R: *Yeah. Well, I mean, you're quite beautiful. Can you take your hijab off? (She does.) Now I can tell you're twelve. It was your eyes that were older. How did you get here?*

C: *We come by illegal way. We come in cars from Iran, then to Pakistan, then to Turkey and then by boat to Greece. It was very hard. Our boat had a hole and it lets in water and we were like all crying. And we took water by our hands to get it out.*

   I saw everything with my eyes. It was so dangerous, really dangerous. It was near to die.

R: *How long were you in the sea?*

C: *I don't know. It was really bad. I was so scared. It was forty-four people and like the boat was size of ping-pong table. The boat is going down and filling with water. My mom had only her head sticking out of water and I was like, 'Help me please.' My mom was under everyone's feet and she was going under. And they take* my mom up. And she was like, 'Thank you. Thank you so much.' She was red. Her skin was really red. She was so scared. And then a boat came.

R: And it rescued you?

C: They come and help us.

R: How would you describe camp life?

C: It's very dangerous. Men are drunk, they fight with knife, they hit each other and they sometimes kill each other. I scared so I sit at home all alone and don't come out.

R: You don't leave home? What do you do all day?

C: I have my phone with me and earphones and I listen to BTS (South Korean K-pop boy band). They make me happy and make me find myself and make me feel I'm alive. It's very bad that you love seven boys from Korea and they don't know that you exist. One day I will go to the concert and one day I will see them. I'm thinking about this every night. I like talking to you.

R: Me too with you.

C: It's so good to talk and say about my life. That's a really good feeling. You know my English not so good. And I should sit and train in home. But when I'm home I say, 'No, who cares about English?' I like to learn Korean because BTS, seven boys are from Korea. I want to live there and meet them. I listen on phone and I dance alone. You know I made the decision last night. I want to write in a notebook all of my dreams and I'm going to make them come true. I will do that. I will go to BTS concert. I will have a good future. I will help my siblings in any problem that they will have. And the last thing that is going to be, I will save somebody *from the death. This is the last dream I have. Like if they knew that that person is going to die, I want to save them. I want to do this one day.*

R: *That's amazing for a twelve-year-old.*

*

I listen to all their dreams knowing, most likely, they won't come true – it's heart-breaking. But it's all they've got. Here's the rub: most people in the camp will never get out. It's a 'Catch-22' situation. If they pass the many interviews, they'll get a tourist visa for some safe country. When they get there, they won't get a job because there aren't any, especially for refugees. The tourist visa will expire six months later and then they'll be sent back to Greece. Refugees who were once teachers, doctors, academics, engineers, lawyers can't get jobs as street sweepers or sewer cleaners in Greece, let alone anywhere else.

I became close friends with a family at the camp. The man was in his early thirties, I'll call him N. He had been a policeman in Afghanistan, and later trained as a lawyer. His wife had been attending her economics class at the university in Kabul when the building was bombed. Probably because there were so many females in her class. The couple had a small child.

I asked if we could trade phone numbers. When I got back to London, N texted me. I received his text while shopping at Peter Jones. I had been, of all things, trying to find a goose feather-filled pillow. I read the beginning of the text as I was squeezing various species of goose pillows. I stopped after a few sentences.

If you can please help my family they are really in Death Danger. I was police officer for 7 Year's in Criminal Deportment the Taliban wanted from me to left my job and work for them but I didn't and after that they was put some letters at our house: 'you are working for foreigners and you are infidels, we have warned you many times to leave your duty and cooperate with us like a real Muslim. but you did not accept and you harmed our Mujahideen. Wait for your death and your family death.'

After some days they armed attack on me. I left I come out from Afghanistan but unfortunately Taliban didn't left my family. They take out my uncle from house and 2 days later my family was received a DVD the Taliban recorded. In that video the Taliban pour oils on my uncle, he was alive they burn and killed him. Also they said we would do worse of this with all of you.

After that my family left Afghanistan and went to Iran. But unfortunately my family was deported from Iran. Now they are really in death danger because my father worked for long time as Deputy Chief of Operations with Foreigners at Mine Clearance company by the name of HALO TRUST in Afghanistan and my sister was main reporter for more than five years on TV News Channel, now they are living in our relatives house and every moment something bad can happen to them. Also you know all and everything about us and our living place we can't do anything just are seeing when they will Die 😭😭

N had no idea who I was or what I did in the UK but he didn't meet many people from the West so he reached out to me. He sent me the ID cards of his five family members who were now in hiding. This is not my turf, getting people out of Afghanistan, so I had no idea what to do.

In another text, he gave me the phone number of someone to call who might be able to help get his family out. Another thing he didn't tell me is that his sister was the leading anchorwoman on the most watched news programme, interviewing some of the most powerful world leaders. Now she's in hiding because being a famous woman (more stress on woman), she'd probably be the highest name on the Taliban hit list.

The four other family members had the word 'HALO' stamped on the photos. The Halo Trust, as it turned out, is a UK humanitarian charity that was supported by Princess Diana. It was founded in Kabul after the Soviets withdrew, leaving behind charming mementos of their visit in the form of landmines. Halo trained its employees to be minesweepers.

I emailed the Halo Trust to tell them some of their employees were still in Afghanistan. Could they please get them out? I got an email back thanking me for my concern, but they'd got everyone out that they could. I wanted to tell them I was a friend of Diana Spencer and how unhappy it would have made her that some employees were left in Afghanistan. Later I thought maybe not a great move.

Then I called the number N gave me. What are the chances of a refugee in Athens connecting me to someone I already know? The person who picked up the phone told me she worked for Helena Kennedy, aka Baroness Kennedy of The Shaws, QC, FRSA, HonFRSE. She's a Scottish barrister, Labour member of the House of Lords, was Principal of Mansfield College, Oxford, and my friend.

Anyway, Helena was incredibly helpful but she was involved in her own missions. Working day and night for the last six months, she had got 200 women judges to safety from Afghanistan. I am in awe of this woman.

I was put in touch with a few people who told me they could help. I was suddenly caught in a spider's web of intrigue and confusion. I spoke to some people who had no experience in rescue operations but wanted to do some good, along with becoming heroes. It was hard to tell if they were doing this out of kindness or if they were caught up in some sort of James Bond fantasy. Or both.

I paid for five passports but never received them because the following day the passport office was bombed by a suicide bomber.

In the end the people who were helping me got the passports at another office. One of the contacts I was in touch with managed to get N and his family out of the refugee camp and into Europe, where he's now safe, has a job and a home. I really just went to fold some clothes and serve tea when I went to the camp – I had no idea it would end with getting him and his family out. I then received this text from N.

Thank you so much dear Respectable Madam. (I have never and never will again be given this title.) Yes we are really happy it's all for your help and kindness to us. You give us new life. I pray that God protects all of yours. 😊🙏😊.

I was in The White Company trying to find a candle called 'Winter'. It has a cinnamon scent that I love. They were out of stock, so I was pissed off and was complaining bitterly to a salesperson when N's next text arrived. After I read it,

I thought I should take the nearest hanger and beat myself for being so self-involved. But maybe it's a good thing to be involved with candles so as not to be faced with the enormity of this new Holocaust, where 22 million people are facing genocide.

> Hello Respectable madam I have to say my family received their passports and did their biometrics. You have really given me the love and joy of a mother. I will be indebted to you as long as I live, I kiss your hands from a distance. I hope my family can safely come out from over there.

Along with the text was a set of photos of each member of the family, proudly and happily holding their newly stamped passports.

N told me that someone had been calling him with updates about getting his family in Afghanistan out and to a safe country. The man mentioned my name but I had no idea who he was. He told N that his family would be evacuated at the end of the month on the next available plane. Then that month came and went. Why not just call and tell him when his family was actually boarding the plane rather than keep him hoping? The man called N again, saying it was still going to happen the next month. That month came and went, too.

Then the contact got in touch with me and said N's family in Afghanistan was at the top of the list to get out. I didn't know this person. It didn't make sense. Why was he calling me with information about this particular family when there are so many families who need to escape? He told me there was going to be a documentary made and would I do a short interview about him? I wondered if maybe this person thought I could get him a little fame, I hope not. I said when you get the family out, I'll talk.

N writes me.

Hi madam, I'm really sorry for annoying you again. Now I received another call from that man who is telling us he's arranging flights.

We also wish that he could do something to save us because my family is really in a very bad situation and all the doors are closed. 😔😔😔

Believe me it is extremely difficult for us to bear all this waiting. Sometimes I feel that my heart is tearing apart. We owe you for all of your kindness. 🙏🙏🙏

Another of my mysterious contacts told me I should pay for the family to get to Pakistan and for their accommodation while they waited to get a US visa. I asked someone I knew in the House of Lords their opinion and received this email.

Dear Ruby,

I think the die is now cast in Afghanistan and getting people out will be increasingly difficult. There was a brief period when evacuations were more possible because the Taliban were not yet deeply embedded. The movement of people went unnoticed or a blind eye was turned. I think now it is much harder and there are more informants, anxious to ingratiate themselves with the new established powers i.e. the Taliban.

I also think that the visa situation is dire. Countries are retreating from their asylum obligations. Governments everywhere fear a backlash from their populations, especially as economic circumstances are becoming so tough in all our countries.

I too continue to receive messages from desperate-sounding people but I tell them honestly that it is no longer possible to get visas. Which is certainly true in Britain. Or I let the message pass.

I think your contact was trying to help but I don't believe it's possible at this time.

I think you have all done God's work in getting people out. Now you have to get back to your own life. There is going to be plenty of good stuff to do here in the months to come.

My advice is to edge away at this stage.

The man is still calling N, pumping him full of new hope with another possible date in the far-off future for his family to get to safety. I spoke to the man today and he told me he has a different country lined up to give the family visas and explained their route to getting there. My opinion is this will never happen, but I'd like to be proved wrong.

Clinic

7 June 2022

Shrink session
The shrink is looking for her notepad. I hope it's not because she can't remember who I am. I pray that I'm her favourite.

S: You told me last week that after Ed watched your daughters per-
form their show, he said they were 'good'. And there was a moment
that generated quite a lot of emotion for you.

I'm thrilled whenever the shrink remembers where we left
off in a session. It shows she does remember who I am.

R: Well, the word 'good' scares me because you need more than
'good' in this business. You have to be excellent and push hard to
get anywhere. I'm terrified that if my kids don't make it, they'll
feel like I did when I was turned down. It almost broke me.

S: Because of the damage your father inflicted, you should
step back from your daughters. They aren't you, and they
weren't tormented. They'll be able to take the successes and
failures more in their stride than you could. Should we do some
EMDR now?

R: Okay.

S: I want you to connect with that memory of when Ed said that
the girls were good. What were the emotions you felt when he said
that? What's the picture in your mind as you follow the ball to the
left and right and back across the screen?

R: In my imagination, one of my daughters is really upset. In my
mind, she looks heartbroken.

S: We're going to work with this. Take the image of your upset
daughter. Where do you feel the fear in your body?

R: In my heart.

S: As you're feeling fear in your heart, what's the belief you have
about yourself?

R: That I wouldn't just have been heartbroken if I didn't make it. I would have gone under. Because not making it would mean I'd be stuck at home forever. I would have killed myself.

S: Take that image of your heartbroken daughter, together with the fear in your heart and the belief that you would kill yourself. Now drop back to childhood. Follow the ball on the screen and tell me the very first place that you land.

R: In my bedroom.

S: Just tell me what you're getting now you've come back to that bedroom. What's coming up?

R: I think I'm more angry now. Yeah. Because I wasn't allowed in my own closet.

S: What are you noticing?

R: My mother put all my underwear in plastic bags and she has piled them up in the order of how old I was when I wore them from around four. She kept them for some reason. All of my clothes are hanging in plastic bags. Nice clothes. We'd go to a shop called Young At Heart and my mother would buy me really expensive dresses, and I hated all of them. She bought so many for me but I don't remember leaving the house so where was I going to wear them?

S: So your mother buys all these amazing clothes and then you don't go anywhere where you could wear them?

R: I don't know, maybe a wedding or something, but I never went to a wedding. My cousin got all my hand-me-downs. But I don't know what was handed down because I never wore them.

S: *So what's coming up?*

R: *I'm confused as to what the clothes were for.*

S: *But just go with the confusion.*

R: *They never gave me a front door key, so if I was let out at night, I'd have to knock on the window. My mother never slept. She's sitting with that dog till four in the morning so she'd let me in. They let me drive their car as long as they knew where I was going. Then they'd both inspect me for signs of drug use. I remember my father going out to our car to collect the ashtray. He wanted me to identify the contents. I'd rake through the heap of ashes going, 'Cigarette butt, gum, gum, gum wrapper, gum, butt, butt, wrapper, etc.' If he suspected a lump of something unidentifiable, he'd break into a tirade of what a 'no good bum' I was. This could end in some sort of punishment like I couldn't leave the house for two weeks. What was the difference, I was locked in anyway. Oh, my God, it just occurred to me – I was never really let out of the house, I was actually a lock-in – I never realized. It was like the kids who were locked in the basement by their father. The guy from Austria. Maybe it's a tradition in Vienna to lock up your daughters.*

S: *Did you have a safe place where you could be by yourself?*

R: *No, my bedroom door didn't lock. Neither did my bathroom door. They could burst through like stormtroopers at any moment. Sometimes my mother would burst into the bathroom, grab my underwear and scrub them hard with soap almost before I took them off. You know, I have dreams that I'm having sex with somebody in the bathroom and my parents break in.*

I have to lie down now. I have to stop.

*

8 June 2022

Recently I've started going to the coffee shop Max found online. Today I discovered I could sit alone among people. I listened to their conversations and instead of the usual envy that I wasn't them, I started to think I was lucky I was on my own, their stories bored me.

*

Clinic

Shrink session

R: I didn't really go out with men until my twenties. My dad would say I was a loser, and that's why no man ever asked me out, but when I finally had a boyfriend in my mid-twenties – I met him in Scotland – my parents helped end it. He promised he'd write to me, but there were never any letters after I got back to Evanston. I was heartbroken. When I cleared up the house after my parents died, I found a file my mother kept hidden from me, with all his letters stuffed into it.

S: She hid his love letters from you?

R: Yes. And because I never heard from him, I assumed the boyfriend had dropped me. Later in my twenties, I was in love with a guy who had that ugly but sexy thing going on. When my father met him, he turned to me in front of him and said, 'This is an atrocity of nature. How could you be with a man like this? Ruby, have you lost your mind?' The guy dumped me on the spot.

Years later I was with my father and Alan Rickman at dinner when my dad suddenly turned to me and said, 'Whatever happened to that loser you went out with?' Alan, who knew the guy, said, 'That loser just sold his production company for sixty million pounds.' My father nearly choked.

I recently asked Rima, Alan Rickman's partner, if she remembers if I went out in the evenings with Alan when he came to stay with my family at their condo in Miami along with some other friends from the RSC. She said Alan always wondered why he'd go out with them but I stayed in. It didn't seem odd to me back then because it was my normal. My parents went on and on about how dangerous it was to go out at night and I finally succumbed without a fight.

I'm such a strong person, I wonder why I didn't just walk out? I suppose the fear of abandonment had something to do with it. I once saw a mother beating her child and afterwards, the child went to the mother. He needed to get hugged by the abuser. I understand that completely.

9 June 2022

The bike fills up my room (I asked Ed to bring it and of course he has) – I finally built up the courage and decided to take it out for a spin. Rule number 1: Don't let a person who is in a mental clinic go out to ride their bike. Of course, as I leave it begins to rain. I mean waterfalls are released on my head, but do I turn around? No, of course not, I'm determined to get where I'm going for coffee. I have to ride down a busy street and I'm splashed by buses, which I'm weaving in and out of.

While I'm taking a turn, I lose my balance and fall over. A few people rush over to help as I'm lying sideways in the street. Cars are swerving around me. I don't want to seem like an old person, so I hear myself say, 'I'm fine. I've done this on purpose, I'm just trying out a new bike.' I've cut my leg and am trying to not let them see I'm bleeding from both knees through my pants.

5

Television

You cannot walk the second half of life's journey with first journey tools. You need a whole new tool kit.

— Richard Rohr

Let me tell you a little about my relationship to television. My father always told me that when I failed in this acting 'nonsense', which was inevitable, he'd set me up with a little linen business in Evanston. The reason I wanted to be on television is because I knew if I could just keep myself on the air, I'd never have to go home. So I bulldozed my way to a career in TV and a regular series that lasted twenty-five years. I toured the world filming documentaries.

I don't remember asking anyone at the BBC for permission, I just filmed year after year. I made a show in a Texas brothel called the Chicken Ranch and filmed the real lives of porno stars. The KKK made me Head Wizard, and I watched as fundamentalist church-goers in Appalachia threw copperheads and rattlesnakes at each other, in the vain hope of proving that God loved them – by not getting bitten. Many congregation members I noticed had missing fingers. I attended beauty pageants for five-year-olds, and I went on a trip to Russia during Glasnost and so many more.

After years of doing documentaries, the BBC asked me to

interview stars. They were called stars in those days rather than celebrities. A celeb can be someone who rolls in off the street wearing a dental-floss-stringed thong, partnered with a couple of air-bag mammaries. A star was someone who had talent, which was once necessary to work on television or film. I thought okay, I'd do a year of interviewing stars and then I'd go back to my beloved documentaries.

I've never been interested in doing interviews sitting at a desk, slinging questions. To avoid being that kind of one-liner gag merchant, I often invited the guests to participate in making the documentaries with me. Carrie Fisher and I went to find her the ideal cowboy while herding and learning to castrate cattle. While interviewing Hugh Hefner at the Playboy mansion, I lived in the bunny dorm with the latest batch of bunnies.

At the BBC there is a rule: 'No jobs for women over fifty.' Just when I thought my best years were ahead of me, I was fired. I had committed the heinous crime of turning five zero, and there are few exceptions to this rule at the BBC. The only time they're prepared to break it is if the budget won't stretch to prosthetics for a twenty-year-old so they need the authentic old one. The other time they use a 'real' old person is for a reality show where they send them to a hospice in India and the viewers can watch them get confused and act dotty. But in general, when an actress hits fifty, she'll be put out to TV pasture and chances are she'll never be heard of again.

Apart from turning fifty, there are other hidden disadvantages. If you're in show business all responsibilities are removed and you live in a world where everything is done for you. Then when the career begins to dip, you're expected to go back to behaving like a normal person. If this person never had to do the simple essentials, like get a coffee or drive somewhere, how would they know how to survive in the world? They're helpless, like a baby. All they ever had to do was point and say, 'Get me that.'

If you're a doctor, plumber, teacher or any other profession, people assume you can feed yourself and get yourself to work on time. In show business there are people hired to make sure there are no stains on your clothes and your hair is combed. Please don't think I'm complaining; it was heaven. I'm just saying the fallout is that you become a junkie to this kind of personal slavery. I was on television for over twenty-five years, getting cups of tea brought to me on a whim, so it was pretty hard for me to get used to the idea of boiling water for myself.

Humans are creatures of habit, and if you keep infantilizing them day after day, they will become entitled and expect to be treated as 'special'. I have seen sensible, educated people throw a hissy fit because they didn't get their latte with the Himalayan yak breast milk they ordered. When I first had to use public transport, out of habit, I would march to the front of the ticket queue and when someone shouted, 'Hey, asshole, get in the line like everyone else,' a pathetic part of me wanted to say, 'Do you know who I am?' I held back or they would have trampled me to death.

I wanted to prove to everyone I wasn't going down with the ship. (The ship being my career.) So I pulled up the throttle and got into Oxford. In retrospect, being fired was a good thing. I've managed to build a life and a more interesting career. Since the firing, I've built a great brain (mine) by learning about the brain. (No matter how mammaried you are, you can't take that from me.) And now that I'm thinking about it, I wouldn't have received an OBE if I hadn't been thrown out of television, so in a strange way I should be grateful it happened, write them a thank you letter.

Clinic

10 June 2022

I go to tea with a friend in the fancy hotel next door. I order scones and tea for two in the hope of communicating 'I may look homeless but I have money.' But I look around and realize no one is looking at me. People aren't saying to each other, 'Isn't that the woman from television?' And 'I wonder why she isn't on it any more.' I'm invisible again, like I was before my career took off. If they did finally recognize me they'd go, 'What the hell happened to her?'

I look like hell, so there's no connection between my made-up TV face and this greenish, tired, Herman Munster one. The good thing about being invisible is, I can watch everyone without being watched.

They say you lose your talent in writing or acting when you become the 'observed' rather than the 'observer'. How can you understand human nature, act it or write about it when you're always scanning the room to see who's looking at you and then getting pissed off because people are staring, and even more pissed off when you notice no one is looking? When you believe the spotlight is on you, you start performing, becoming the personality they want you to be to keep them loving you. You perform because you don't want to disappoint, in case they find out you're really a boring person or just a person. It's exhausting. Now I can stare all I want at anybody and no one stares back. What bliss. I arrive at the clinic, doors whoosh open, I walk upstairs and line up for my meds, which is part of my routine. I register a flicker of joy because I'm surrounded by my people, I'm drugged and there's crap food, so I'm losing weight.

11 June 2022

Shrink session

R: *I survived by building a career in television. Though my parents were repeatedly telling me what a disappointment I was in looks, brains and personality, I reinvented myself almost overnight. I learned to be funny. I honed it, took it to the UK and sold it as television fodder. I achieved what my parents couldn't – the American Dream.*

S: *Can you remember the first time you learned that you were funny and could use it?*

R: *I don't remember the exact moment, just that it happened in my final year of high school. It came out one day, like being possessed by Joan Rivers. As soon as I learned to speak comedy, I attracted the boys. Not just the boys, I got the 'Golden God of High School', the star of the football team. Of course I didn't know he was gay, but neither did he. And because he liked me, all the popular girls suddenly wanted me to be their newest 'bestie'. Now I was the 'it' girl like my mother was.*

S: *You learned that you could engage people, attract them through your humour. Because you didn't get that love, you had to find a way of getting it.*

R: *Where that went wrong was that it became an addiction. I became insatiable to get a bigger crowd around me.*

*

I'm being a little extreme about not being offered anything on television. I was asked to do *Stars – Dancing on Ice*. Or in my case, 'Stars – falling over and breaking their heads open'. I also had an interesting offer for a documentary series that I'd like to share with you. I want to say from the start, I am not making this up. What you are about to read is completely true.

I had just done a book and a tour all over the UK with a monk, Gelong Thubten, and a neuroscientist, Ash Ranpura, talking about the brain and the mind, called *How to be Human*. A producer had seen it, loved it and sent me the following proposal. It was for a series he created just for us called, 'All Aboard the Life Coach'. I hope you'll enjoy this as much as I did.

The show would involve the three of us arranging bus tours to help mentally ill people. The first sentence of the proposal went, 'What do you get when you cross a neuroscientist, a Buddhist monk and Ruby Wax? One hell of a road trip!' It continues, 'Not only do the people on the bus have mental illness but so does the crew, from the cameramen to the makeup artist and perhaps even the driver. There will be the usual bumps along the road: Thubten (the monk) is stuck in charge of changing a flat tyre on the bus; Ruby is dealing with a travel-sick holiday-maker, whilst Dr Ash is facing language barriers trying to order the group's lunch.'

This is one of my favourite parts: 'There may be times when it becomes too much for the production team and Ruby needs to take control of the camera to keep it rolling.'

What were they thinking? That the cameraman might have a mental breakdown and just curl up in a bush somewhere and I have to learn how to film the show while he's

taken away to a mental institution? Then maybe the sound-
man takes an overdose? So the monk is now on sound while
Ash learns to do makeup?

'PLACES THEY WILL GO.

They take the mentally ill people to Bali where learning to
surf among the breathtaking scenery helps ease their mental
suffering. They will also attend a NGaben ceremony, a cele-
bration of death.'

'Next they bring the mentally ill passengers to Botswana
where they try the local medicine man's treatment for
depression – staying up all night and then killing a chicken to
eat for breakfast. They will also take part in a "Colossal Purifi-
cation Ceremony". It will be an incredible journey that will
lift the hearts of all involved.'

I started to think this might be a genius comedy idea and
missed my chance.

Okay, I thought, that's my farewell to show business, but
no, around the same time that I was organizing my journeys
for this 'finding meaning' book, I was offered another documentary series. More about that later. Now you may think
after my experiences in revisiting my career, I would turn the
offer down. I didn't. Fame is very addictive and mama needs
new shoes. When the siren song of television calls me back to
visit its shores, the old craving for approval rears its head. I'm
reminded of when Sally Field shrieked at the audience at the
Oscars, 'You like me! You like me!'

Here's how it all started. A member of the team who
works for Louis Theroux (he has a team to dial the phone,
like I once did) called to ask if I could do an interview. I
assumed Louis Theroux had been my replacement. In my
paranoid mind he had not only snatched my career but had

taken food from my children's mouths. This triggered something very primal in me. After I was fired, he became my nemesis. I've never seen his shows, nor did I allow my children to watch them.

Putting all that aside, I told them, okay, I'd do his podcast. It wasn't for a few months. But you know when you say you'll do something in a few months and then suddenly those few months are up? That's what happened to me. At the time I was staying in Findhorn for a break, an eco community in Scotland for people who want to live an alternative lifestyle while not fucking up the planet. I wrote about Findhorn in my last book. (You can look it up by simply buying it.) I stayed above a healing centre. When I mentioned to a couple of the healers that I was sick with anxiety because I was going to have an interview with Louis Theroux and I was afraid I wouldn't be able to speak, they offered to help. Next thing I knew, they were laying hands on me to calm me down. Many hands. I fell into a deep sleep and woke up at 7.30am when I heard the same healers knocking on my door offering me more hands on during the interview. This was an offer I couldn't refuse. So when the phone rang, I was ready. The healing had begun.

Louis began the interview by saying he heard I told people not to mention his name or I would vomit. Now, that's not a good intro. In the past I would have tried to crack a joke, which might have offended Louis even more. But with the help of the many healing hands upon me, when I spoke to Louis a very centred, mature, authentic human came out of my mouth.

I confessed to him that I had been under the impression he had taken my job from me. To make matters worse, I told him that about twenty years ago I stood on a stage and had to say, nearly choking with heartbreak, 'And for the best documentary show on television, it's Louis Theroux.' I had to give him not one but two BAFTAs. And that's when I felt like vomiting, I said.

To prepare for the interview, I had watched one of his shows after I got up that morning. I told him that in many ways I thought he was much better than I was. It was clever how he held his cards close to him to give the guests a chance to expose themselves. I, on the other hand, thought I sometimes tried too hard to get them to like me. I was a bit like an over-excited schoolgirl. I told Louis I liked his style and he told me he liked mine. The healers removed their hands. I was fine on my own.

I told him I created my persona out of nerves, but didn't like it, it wasn't really me. (On the other hand, I got 11 million viewers for some shows so maybe it wasn't so bad.)

Louis said he liked how honest I was with my guests, especially when I interviewed Trump. I said it was the worst interview I ever did because he frightened me.

Louis insisted it was a great strategy to show him my vulnerability. I didn't think I was vulnerable at all, I started asking idiotic questions, which I do when someone scares me, especially a powerful man. Then to defend myself I become passive aggressive.

Louis asked me, 'You remember what Trump said? He said, "I can tell you're angry but you're angry with a smile."' I told him Donald had my number, he got me exactly when he said that. He totally deflated me with that observation.

Louis said the BBC should do a compilation of my series. 'Why haven't they done it before?' I confessed I did find it upsetting that no one has ever repeated any of my shows. There are repeats of obscure shows about things like where dogs in Scotland go to the loo, but not my shows.

He turned out to be one of the nicest people I've met in the world of television. The interview went on for about three hours and by the end, we had bonded. Louis emailed me several times telling me he was pushing to get my shows back on the air. How generous was that? I honestly didn't want him to push it but he did anyway. The outcome was they showed a compilation of my best shows. I was in the studio for days, talking about what I thought about my interviews. Watching my shows while saying what I was thinking at the time to the camera, was a bit like doing my own obituary. Usually someone else talks about your career after you've died, but here was me talking about mine while I was still alive.

My first thought while watching the old interviews was, 'Why didn't anyone tell me how cute I was?' I had a scene in the jacuzzi with Goldie Hawn. I stepped into the water clutching a bathrobe to hide my body. What was I thinking? It wasn't bad at all. Not like Goldie's, which was exercised to the hilt, day and night, but mine was fine. At the age I am now, I should pose naked for a photograph so when I'm ninety-five and I see myself I'll think, 'Wow! What a body!'

As I watched my old interviews, I remembered what a kick it was to make them, how much fun I had and how happy I was. Pamela Anderson let me play her body double while filming *Baywatch*. I changed into a swimsuit and pretended I had cut myself by accident while shaving my legs so there were bits of toilet paper hanging off my inner thighs when I came on the set. It made her laugh, so she played along with the joke and let me do a second show with her. This time we were both in the back seat of a limo while she happily demonstrated her favourite sexual positions on me. I got very confused, it was like genital origami.

I always research my guests, so I knew Bette Midler had worked in a factory stuffing pineapples into tin cans. She'd been doing back-to-back interviews and was tired, so her PR told me I had five minutes with her. By coincidence, I'd also worked in a factory, stuffing onions into the behinds of frozen chickens. (Not easy without pliers.) Bette and I competed over who had the worst job. I let her win. If you show someone a good time they want to stick around and do more, so we took off for Harvey Nichols and ended up in the fish department, where we performed a puppet show using a trout and a halibut. After that she was relaxed and happy enough to go down the escalator singing her latest hits while I stole clothes from the racks behind her. We're friends to this day.

Same thing happened with Jim Carrey. He didn't want to do more than a few minutes. He was also exhausted from a day of interviews for his new film. But we had booked a room at the Dorchester Hotel. We laid out a Royal Doulton china tea service on the dining table. It was all very elaborate and there were many delicate pieces. I encouraged him to do his famous magic act, which would involve pulling the tablecloth from under the tea set. I didn't expect it to work, so I hid behind a sofa. When he pulled out the tablecloth, every item on the table got smashed, the ceiling was splattered in tea, and cream from the scones was smeared into the carpet. The cleaning bill cost a fortune but from that moment on, he went to town. Once Jim realized this was more comedy improvisation than interview, we played for three more hours. Working with him was like lobbing balls to a tennis pro. I'd throw him a feed line and he'd whack back some brilliant retort. Eventually I couldn't get rid of him. He kept trying to get back into the hotel room, pretending to be room service.

John McEnroe let me beat him at tennis when we were in New York. The following week at Wimbledon, I went to interview him on Court One. Apparently it's against the law to step on to a grass tennis court during Wimbledon. No one told me that. So when I walked on to the court, I was immediately arrested and carried away by the police. The incident was discussed in Parliament and the BBC was seriously condemned. I didn't get in trouble, but they did. I'm still friends with John and his wife, Patty.

I suggested to Sharon Stone that we go to a deli to continue our interview. She said she didn't want to be recognized but I had brought Hasidic costumes for us to wear in case she agreed. She liked the idea and went along with it. We spent the afternoon sitting at a counter in our beards and yarmulkes. No one recognized her.

When Sandra Bullock told me what a great waitress she was, I went into my compete mode. She may be a better actress than me but I'm a far greater waitress. Sandra and I decided that to find out who was the better server we'd do a 'waitress-off' and let the customers in a coffee shop vote on it. I am a better waitress but I let her win.

I lay in bed with Madonna. There was not much comedy during the interview, so when she left to go to the loo, to bump it up, I went through her handbag, found a pair of underwear and put them on my head. (I was desperate for something to be funny in the show.) When she came back, she was not amused. We did not exchange phone numbers.

Someone else who really didn't like me was Bill Cosby. At the time of the interview, he was playing the kindly, wise Dr Huxtable in *The Cosby Show* and getting 44.4 million viewers. As soon as he walked in and saw me, he grabbed me around the neck and dragged me into his office off the set. I was made to sit at his feet and address him as Doctor Cosby. Whenever I'd ask him a question, he'd pick up a (real) phone and tell some non-existent person he wanted me removed. Each time I spoke, he would call this invisible person and complain I was useless, and why was it taking them so long to get rid of me. It was a toxic interview. I had a rictus smile on my face throughout. If anyone had watched my TV inter-view with Bill Cosby, they would have spotted this man was dangerous.

While Roseanne Barr was giving me a tour of her lavish house, she took me into a room packed with rag dolls. Her face was sewn on to all of them. She then dressed me up as a bride for some reason when we were going through her closet. At the end of the interview, we got into her bathtub. That's when she told me she was a glutton. She said she couldn't stop shopping or eating. I said to her, 'Because you're a big pig.' I heard a sharp inhale from the crew. They were frightened I had gone too far. They were obviously relieved when Roseanne burst out laughing. At that point, they knew it was going to be fine.

Goldie Hawn and I did the interview under the covers of her hotel bed. We made each other pee from laughing so hard. These days whenever we meet, based on our first encounter, we address each other as 'pee sisters'.

And best but not least was Carrie Fisher. I'd always loved her, not just for Princess Leia, but for her writing. Her books were genius. You want dark? Read *Postcards from the Edge* and be shocked and hysterical simultaneously.

I'd begged my producer to get Carrie Fisher on my show for years, without success. Until finally the day came when Carrie was in the UK and agreed. Naturally I was determined to make her my best friend for life. No pressure there.

During the interview I told her that our fathers had met back in the 1960s. When I was about ten years old, my family took a trip to Las Vegas. Eddie Fisher, a famous crooner in the 50s and 60s, was married to Elizabeth Taylor at the time.

Eddie was sitting with his cronies in the lobby of our hotel, when my father went up to him and said, 'Boy, have I got a beautiful woman for you. You've never seen anything so gorgeous! Come on out here, Ruby.' I was hiding behind a pillar. He shouted for me to come out as he built up a picture of the sexy girl he was going to introduce Eddie Fisher to. I didn't move. Then my mother came up behind me and pushed me out so Eddie and his cronies could see me. They all had a good laugh. I was not an attractive child.

That's how Carrie came to fall for me, because we shared humiliation. When you watch the interview, it's as if you witness a love affair blossom between us. After many years of sharing a bed with Carrie as friends – we travelled together – she suggested I write a book about my parents. Carrie helped me edit it. When she first read it she said my parents were almost as crazy as hers. You could get no finer review. Eddie was a heroin addict and her mother, the legendary Debbie Reynolds of *Singing in the Rain* fame, was publicly humiliated when Eddie ran off with Elizabeth Taylor. I called the book *How Do You Want Me?*

Other highlights? Well, there was the time OJ tried to stab me with a banana (google it and watch with astonishment). We did the interview in a white van identical to the van he made his famous escape in, pursued by helicopters and legions of cop cars. I tried to book us a place for lunch, but when I said it was a table for OJ, the maître d' hung up, so we had to stay in the van for the day. We only got out once. When we went for a walk on Venice Beach, someone approached OJ and said, 'Can I shake the hand of a murderer?' OJ didn't mind. Fame is fame and he loves being the centre of attention even if it's infamy.

Later that night OJ pretended to stab me with a banana. It was about 3am. (I tried to tire him out so he'd lose his defences.) For some reason he thought it would be appropriate to knock on the door of the hotel room we were in from the hallway and pretend to stab me many times with a piece of fruit. His agent wanted to cover up the incident, so he told me, 'OJ's such a kidder. He likes to imitate his favourite films.' I said, '*Psycho*?' The agent said, '*Cats*.' I have never figured out the connection. A short time later, the agent offered to show me where the knife was buried. I backed away.

Another highlight for me was interviewing Imelda Marcos. When her husband was president of the Philippines, 17 billion dollars went missing from the country's coffers. Imelda explained where she found it. Apparently when she was dusting the walls one day, she knocked down a painting. When she removed the exposed nail she saw a glint of gold. Mrs Marcos said it turned out that their entire house had been made out of gold bullion. It was a miracle. Then she changed into her wedding gown and sang over fifteen songs to me. The one I remember most was 'Feelings'.

By a strange coincidence, when I went to throw something in the trash, I saw a copy of *Hello* magazine, with my face on the cover. I have no idea how that particular magazine ended up in the trash, but as soon as I retrieved it and showed it to Imelda she became my biggest fan. As soon as she realized I was famous, she took me to Parliament and announced to the members that I was on the cover of *Hello*. This announcement was followed by a party, where she put me on her lap and fed me chocolate cake. In her excitement

Imelda took me up to her attic and showed me her new stash of shoes. There were thousands of them. But not even close to the 30,000 pairs that were taken by the police when she was arrested during her husband's reign many years earlier. They are now housed in a museum.

Also unforgettable is my biggest car crash: the interview I did with Donald Trump on his private jet. When he told me he wanted to be president of the United States, I laughed, thinking he had a wonderful sense of humour. If I had shut up and let the man talk, maybe he would have hung himself, but I thought he was joking. After I asked him a rather stupid question, he'd had it with me. He told the cameraman to turn the camera off, and demanded that the pilot land the plane immediately. My crew and I were dumped in the middle of Arkansas (Trumpster country). But after we rented a car to travel through different states in search of him, the show really took off. If he hadn't abandoned us in the middle of nowhere, we would never have seen a shooting range with Saddam Hussein's face on the target, let alone discovered the poor man's version of Las Vegas, a place called Branson.

The town of Branson is a newly built replica of America in the 1950s, like the set for *Happy Days*. The shopkeepers were dressed in 50s outfits. I think some of the shopkeepers were confused as to what people wore in the 50s because they were in cowboy costumes, some in Victorian dress, some in bathrobes. Busloads of 'Early Man', who still haven't learnt to get up off all fours and stand erect, go there for their holidays. There they can view some of the saddest acts in the known Universe. The stars perform four times a day because some audience members can't remember if they've seen the show before or not. A rabbi riding on a mule sang Yiddish songs. A woman dressed up as a baby sang about her daddy (who was dead) to a pillow with his face drawn on it, and insisted we all sing along to the chorus, 'Daddy, daddy, there will never be another daddy . . .' I will never forget the sight of Siamese twins making toffee in a candy shop. The attached girls were in pink frilly aprons with four cutesy pigtails. They happily stretched the sugar goo as far as it would go, and as far as they could stretch themselves; and then they'd come together to fold it in. It was mesmerizing, but we were looking for Donald so I had to tear myself away.

We visited a lot more of these all-American tourist holes until we finally caught up with Trump in Atlantic City. He was at Trump Casino to judge a beauty contest. Donald still hated me, but his sidekick Roger Stone probably sensed I was as crazy as he was, because he started to like me. We both watched Donald being mobbed by autograph hunters. These Trump fans wanted Donald to sign his book, which they had to pay a fortune for. This took place in a room called 'The Millionaires' Room'. It was so named because only people who had lost over $10,000 in Trump's casino were allowed to enter. He made them buy his book after fleecing them blind. I was getting a sneak preview of his future voters.

I later met Melania, who was still a lingerie model at the time. I think she was wearing one of her nighties. She told me she found Donald incredibly sexy and that he was not lacking in talent in the bed department. She was a sweet woman, beautiful, and I liked her honesty.

Anyway, in the end I might have won over the Big T because he offered me a lift back to the hotel in his limo. No cameras or sound equipment were allowed in the car. This turned out to be a shame. I thought if people heard the sleaze he spewed about women, they might not have voted for him. Then again how stupid was that? It would only have increased his votes.

12 June 2022

Shrink session

S: *The part of you that was so driven to succeed is what got 'the younger you' out of her pain. But I think one of the things causing difficulty in your life is that now, when that kind of fiercely driven part of you takes control to avoid pain, it only creates more pain.*

R: *Do you think if I didn't have to survive I would have been able to do what I did?*

S: *I don't know. We can only conjecture about the part the younger Ruby played in propelling the older Ruby forwards. Lots of people have talent, but they're not driven to succeed. It's not such a bad thing that some pain motivates you to succeed. It's only unhelpful when it sabotages other areas of your life.*

R: *When I'm back on television, I start to feel the driven part taking over again. No more Ms Nice Guy. I became driven again when the BBC compilation show ended. I was phoning my agent all the time whimpering, 'Did anyone call about work for me?'*

S: *Perhaps it reminded you of your childhood when you felt power-less and at the mercy of your father.*

R: *I always wanted him to know that I was worthwhile even though he gave up on me.*

S: *You've convinced yourself that you've done this all to show your father. But have you shown yourself? Are you convinced that you're worthwhile?*

R: *No, I get people to make me feel I'm worthwhile. I lure them in by being funny. Do you think that's a sort of adaptive survival response?*

S: *Yes. A great injustice was done to you, which is you were never taught by your parents that you were valuable in your own right. In that brilliant book he wrote called* Us, *Terry Real says there's a part of us that 'holds the wound'. He says it developed to protect us from feeling the pain of the wound. I think for you, the wound is your feeling of being trapped, alone and unlovable. And the part of you that holds the wound has been telling you, 'I have to succeed because I can't get out of this pain without striving hard.' Terry Real believes it's important that we use our wiser adult mind to work out if the parts that drove us early in life are useful to us in the present.*

R: *Can we stop now? I'm so tired from all this thinking.*

★

After my compilation was aired, strangers started stopping me in the street, telling me how much they loved the show and asking why I wasn't on television any more.

I was beginning to think I had been pretty good at interviewing. There was so much attention that I could feel the old ego stirring. I was regaining my confidence, along with a smidge of arrogance. That's usually when karma comes to kick me in the ass.

So, what happened next, you ask? I never heard from the BBC or anyone again. No phone calls to say 'hi', no commission for another show, nada. So, there it was, an emotional rerun of the first kick in the teeth fifteen years earlier. Back then I was told that the distribution company for the BBC wasn't backing my shows any more because people weren't watching them. This turned out to be a lie. I found out later that a very powerful executive at the time wanted my time slot and so just went in there and took it. I shall not name names.

I'd like to say I wasn't bothered by being rejected again but I'd be lying. It wasn't as bad as the first time, when I ended up with a depression the size of South America. Back then it took me five months to return to the living. But I did feel slightly ashamed that I fell for the old lure of fame, like a moth to a flame.

So what happened next? I was offered that documentary series I was talking about. The not so good news? It would start filming three days after Ed and I got back from the Dominican Republic.

The obvious answer was No. The timing was all wrong. Did I say No? I couldn't. Why? Because the series was going to follow the footsteps of Isabella Bird – who is my heroine! I accepted. In my opinion, Isabella Bird lit the fuse to the dynamite that exploded into the feminist movement. Your options as a woman back then were baking cakes, breeding or being a factory worker. Isabella was a Victorian explorer.

In the 1900s she set off from Yorkshire, aged forty-two, to travel the world. Despite the fact she was still suffering chronic pain from an operation to remove a tumour on her spine (without anaesthesia!), she crossed 800 miles of the Rockies on horseback. Next to her, we are all wimps.

I'm pretty sure she wasn't doing the trip for the purpose of finding meaning. She wanted the scenery to keep changing. She tried to distract herself from the physical and mental trauma she'd been through. I could identify with that.

After she crossed the Rockies, she kept moving. Isabella

toured through Hawaii, Australia, New Zealand, the Middle East, India, China and Japan until she finally galloped across Morocco in her late sixties. Her back still hurt, but you can't say she didn't try to outride the pain.

When the production company asked me to do the show I agreed immediately. I'd be travelling with someone I'd always loved: Mel B from the Spice Girls. My kids used to dress up like her. In their opinion, the most impressive thing I've ever done in my career is interviewing the Spice Girls. My other travel companion would be the actress and comedian Emily Atack. I hadn't heard of Emily because she's only thirty-two, so to me she wasn't born yet.

The idea behind the project was that we would follow in Isabella's footsteps. On horseback. The brief said the three of us would be going mountain climbing, skiing, fly fishing, kayaking and snowshoeing. Outdoors activities for the extremely butch at heart.

Ed thought it was a great idea as long as it didn't turn out to be a reality show about three women competing against each other in the wild, and then, due to impending starvation, making the audience choose which one of us we should eat. I told the production company that I would only do the show if it was an homage to Isabella Bird, not some gladiatorial competition between me, Mel B and Emily.

11 April 2022

We landed in Denver. It wasn't at all how I remembered it from when I went to university there. Denver used to be a hick town filled with run-down bars and junk shops. Now it was a shopping mall, with those old, tired generic shops identical in every American town and city.

To get through university I worked at a strip bar called, 'Sid King's Crazy Horse Bar'. I served cocktails to the customers, and with my saucy (borderline abusive) banter, made a fortune in tips. The strippers were bored with their tired old routines. Some of them complained to me, and I offered to direct them in a Chekhov play. When the strippers performed it before the customers one night, the boss was not happy. I was fired shortly after opening night. Now I was back in town, and making a TV show. Who would have ever dreamt this?

Yes, those were the days. I remember a party where my friends and I got stoned. We decided to go to the Chinese restaurant around the corner and release all the lobsters from their tank as a protest against animal cruelty. Sadly they were squished by oncoming traffic but I still wanted to show Emily and Mel the actual spot where I released them.

13 April 2022

The first morning of shooting I watched as Mel and Emily were being plucked, primped and painted, and turned into ravishing beauties. I expected to look similar after I had my makeup and hair done. The makeup guy kept telling me, 'You're gorge, absolutely gorge!' to build up my 'below the floorboards' self-esteem. But when he finally held up the mirror, there I was: a sagging, crinkled old alligator. I hid my face behind my hand like in *Phantom of the Opera* and begged the makeup guy, 'More concealer!' God bless him, he did what he could, but the crinkles were like deep cracks in the Grand Canyon, and they only got deeper.

When I was young, I looked great at every angle I was

photographed from. Now there's only one angle I can look good from and that's if the camera is glued on the ceiling. I'm not happy about ageing. I expect very few people are, but I'm not them, so it's worse for me.

It was day one, and the director asked each of us to talk into the camera about why we came on this trip. I started talking about Isabella's book, *A Lady's Life in the Rocky Mountains*, and why I loved it. When I was met with blank faces, I realized not many people had read the book.

Our first location was a saloon. It was somewhere close to Cheyenne, the town where Isabella had started her journey, so we seemed to be on the right track. The bar resembled an abattoir: dead stuffed animals everywhere – raccoons, moose, buffalo, coyotes, deer, bear . . . all of nature was hanging on the walls, but stuffed. Name an animal, any animal, they were up there. Attenborough would have had a heart attack.

When the bar keeper came to take our order, she told us about this place being inhabited by ghosts and how if you listen you can hear scratching coming from the inside of the freezer.

The owner served us 'Rocky Mountain oysters'. She said they were the specialty of the house. Emily was first to try one. She told us it was tough, impossible to swallow. When Emily asked what it was she was chewing, the woman, with a big smirk on her face, said, 'Bull's bollocks.' God bless Emily, she kept right on chewing. She's a pro.

14 April 2022

The next day we drove to Cheyenne, which had been Isabella's first stop. We passed a poster in the window of a run-down bar announcing 'comedy club night'. It had a photo of a woman sitting on the toilet. The date had already passed. There was a strip club with a sign 'Open 24 hours a day'. While the crew was setting up, I decided I had to check it out. I tried to get Mel to come and see the show with me, but sensibly she refused. The strip club was a shed. Inside there were withered, seriously pissed go-go dancers clutching a pole with their nicotine-stained fingers. You could hear the cracks as they tried to kick up an old arthritic leg. This town seemed to have nothing much going for it.

For the first set-up, we were taken to some wrangler shop to select our cowgirl clothes. It's hard to make a scene entertaining when you're just picking out a cowboy hat, so I ended up bouncing on a large inflatable rubber ball with horns on it representing a bull. This is why television can bring out the worst in me. I get this overwhelming desire to be funny, even if there's nothing funny going on and it becomes desperate and pathetic. Mel and Emily were embarrassed for me. I could tell.

15 April 2022

We were staying at a dude ranch in the heart of the Rockies where Isabella once spent the night. Today we were told we were going to be on horseback so we could follow the trail Isabella rode on. In the first scene we got introduced to our horses. I showed off my skill in horse-whispering, a gift I claimed I was born with. I was actually stage-whispering some little-known facts about Isabella I wanted to sneak into the film.

The director told us to mount our horses. Mel, as it turns out, couldn't ride. Though she tried to look like she was a pro, her horse knew better, and insisted on taking her in the opposite direction. Mel shouted at me. She accused me of throwing a curse on her horse while I was whispering up its nose.

Mel and I had a very abusive/loving relationship going for us. In every scene we had, she'd insist I had no idea what I was talking about. And vice versa. We flirted through our bickering – that's how women do it. She brushed aside any compliments about her contribution to the Spice Girls' global popularity. She didn't seem to grasp how influential the band had been for an entire generation. It was the first time a girl band whipped the ass of boy bands. There was no doubt she'd achieved huge success, but sadly not in the area of her equestrian skills, which were nil.

In the afternoon, we were going to learn to herd cattle, which I thought might be a good skill to have up my sleeve. Isabella had wrangled thousands of cattle across the plains to make money. We watched two cowgirls demonstrate how to steer twenty calves out of the corral and into the open fields. Unfortunately neither of them was succeeding, so filming halted. Then, seeing the problem, Emily put her iPhone down. She walked over to the corral, and casually trotted the twenty calves out into the fields. Then she picked up the iPhone and continued where she had left off, snapping selfies.

16 April 2022

We were driven out to Knotty Ridge. This was to be a practice run for the final scene of the series when we were informed the three of us would climb Pikes Peak, coming in at 15,000 feet, like Isabella did. When I saw it was a climb up a sheer cliff, I thought, 'Oh no, this isn't about Isabella Bird, we're doing a kind of, "Help Me I'm a Celebrity" thing to see which one of us survives.'

I called Ed and said, 'Help me, I'm a celebrity, get me out of here.' He told me to just keep talking about Isabella.

Our mountain instructor looked like a Ken doll, all chiselled with teeth. He said into the camera in a patronizing tone of voice, 'Come on, Ruby, you'll make it. I've got ya, I promise I'll get you up. I lift hundred pound weights so you should be light as a feather.' Ken tied a rope harness around me and under me. When we got to the cliff face, he tried to pull me up by the rope harness but all I got from all his heaving was a camel toe.

Emily refused the rope harness. She started dragging herself up the smooth rock face by her fake acrylic nails. She was shrieking from the pain, but God damn it, she got to the top of the mountain.

I snapped photos of Emily's ascent from the bottom, and that angle probably got her another million viewers. Then, not to be outdone, Mel started rock climbing straight up in her leopard print onesie. Competitive? You think? This show was intended to be about one woman with balls, but I was working with two.

17 April 2022

For lunch we went to a restaurant which resembled an ol' Western log cabin. It was called 'Bird and Jim', as an homage to Isabella Bird and Mountain Jim. I'll tell you more about him later. We sat down at a rickety wooden table. Our waitress was trying unsuccessfully to hold the pen while taking our orders. She was missing most of her fingers, so of course

I had to ask why. She told us she was electrocuted during a power surge. At the time she was holding an electric drill and carving a flower into the very table we were sitting at. She remembered she was lying on the floor, knowing she was dying. She saw herself in a thick forest. Ahead of her there was a tunnel, and dark figures were beckoning her to go through. She approached the tunnel, but then at the last second, she refused to enter. After she woke up and struggled to her feet, she managed to sew a few of her fingers back on. Then she asked us if we'd decided what we wanted for lunch. We were supposed to order food after that?

Later in the afternoon, we met Tim, a rugged silver fox of a cowboy. He lives on the top of a mountain and only comes down to get supplies. I imagined him to be the doppelgänger of Mountain Jim. Isabella described Jim as a desperado, with half his face mauled by a grizzly bear, the other half gorgeous. He'd killed a few men in his time and spent a lot of his nights brawling and kicking ass in saloons. They say she had a romance with him but we'll never know. In the end he was shot in a gunfight.

Mountain Tim turned out to be far more eccentric than meets the eye. He told us in a very nonchalant way that he sold his wife for a horse and now he lives alone. He invited us up to his home, and he took us there vertically in his snowmobile. While he was teaching Emily how to chop logs outside, Mel and I snuck into his bedroom to see if he really lived alone. Maybe he was kidding about selling his wife. We hadn't seen a horse. Then to our horror we heard him coming up the stairs, so we hid. Mel was under the desk and I hid in the closet. Mel was easy to find. He could see her clearly, crouched under the desk, trying her best to look invisible. She explained she was just looking for her earring. Then she pointed to the closet.

When he opened it, I strolled out saying, 'I found your earring, Mel.' It made no sense. There was no earring. But luckily he didn't get mad. The evening ended with us all sitting around the firepit talking about life, and how whatever age you are, you still don't feel you have got it right. Mel suggested we write down on paper what we wanted to get rid of about ourselves and throw it into the fire. I wrote 'envy'.

In the afternoon, we drove through magnificent 10,000-foot mountains with rushing rivers on either side of the road. The walls of the mountains were rose, aqua, emerald green, and they were shining in the sun like precious jewels. Intermittent waterfalls were smashing down the rocks. I felt an urge to get out of the car and see if there was a cabin for sale along the road, but I forced myself to stay put.

We arrived in a hippie town that seemed to specialize in selling things I had thrown out in the 70s, like my lava lamps, damp fake fur coats, occult earrings, stained bell-bottoms and wall-to-wall crystals. Just on the outskirts of town there was a sign that read, 'Cryogenics only 500 yards. Drop in.' Well, this is the kind of weird stuff I loved filming in my documentary days. We arrived at a huge mound of rubbish with a shack on top of it. There was a sign that read 'Kriogentics'. The owner of the misspelt cryogenic service burst out of the entrance: a giant in full lumberjack wear, a hunter's hat and a macabre grin. He welcomed all of us with bear hugs. He told us that business was slow. So far, he only had one customer lying in his freezer. When we asked how he got into the cryogenics business in the first place, he gave us the back story.

It had all started when a Norwegian guy wanted to find somewhere to freeze his grandfather. The idea was to keep him frozen until they'd found a cure for heart attacks. (I would have said, 'Don't hold your breath.') After that, the grandfather would be defrosted and all would be well. It's illegal in Norway to freeze someone, so the young man came to the Wild West looking for a place where someone could ice Grandad on a regular basis and by chance he met this guy, who sold weed by day (it's legal in Colorado). The weed dealer had no background in this area but when the Norwegian offered him fifty dollars an hour, he jumped at it. So every two weeks he opens the freezer and tosses some dry ice over the body. I loved this scene because he let me help him toss ice as he told me about his life. This could be one of my favourite scenes in the series.

When I called Ed to tell him about the cryogenics man, he said he could hear how happy I was. I was with my people at last.

18 April 2022

Today we were driven to Gulch End, an authentic one-street town, unchanged since the 1900s. It's the real deal, with wooden walkways lining a dirt road, an old General Store selling snake oil and those swinging saloon doors. It was the first place the early settlers panned for gold. People came from all over America to stake their claim to make themselves rich. One gold panner became a billionaire; everyone else left as poor as they came.

Hippies took Gulch End over in the 60s, and Stills, of Crosby, Stills & Nash, lived here. They'd play regular gigs on Friday nights.

Okay, I know you must be sick of it, but I really wanted to live in Gulch End. I couldn't help myself, I called Ed. He hung up.

Today, the whole population seemed to be in the bar, throwin' it back. The specialty of the house was gin and pickle juice. The boys in the bar loved Mel so much we got free pickle juice gins. We danced the night away, being flipped in the air and dragged by our hair on the floor. They told us that's how they dance in Colorado.

This is the America I love; raw and real. I would have never left if it was all like this, but then I would have had to come a century ago.

19 April 2022

Today we visited Central City, the capital of the US in 1831. Ulysses S. Grant – he was the one who thought of turning gold into dollars – stayed there at the swankiest hotel not just in town but in the whole United States. We ran into the Mayor. He told us it would be a dream come true to turn Central City back to the old days. I wanted to say, 'Don't count on it.'

Formerly the pride of America with a famous theatre and wall-to-wall saloons, today the saloons have been replaced by seedy wall-to-wall gambling houses where desperate people sit all day smoking and playing the one-armed bandits, their only exercise being the arm that is moving the lever up and down, as they spend their last dime trying to get three apples in a row.

From Central City we drove to a new location. This one appeared to be a ghost town. There were empty buildings everywhere. I thought people must have left in a rush because of something terrible that was happening. Rocking chairs seemed to still be rocking and the doors still creaking. Mel and Emily were given detectors to pan for gold. While they wasted their time – they only found a belt buckle and a bullet – I interviewed a local expert. He told me that after someone found a gold vein, the town's population went from 10,000 to 100,000 almost overnight. The mining continued for ten years, until eventually there was a hole in the mountain the size of the Grand Canyon. There was nothing left: no trees, no plants, just dusty soil. The land was devastated.

I couldn't help but think it's how we're leaving the whole planet today.

Then suddenly every member of the crew put their equipment down and turned towards me. Someone brought out a cake and the crew started singing 'Happy Birthday'. They must have taken a wild guess how old I was because there were about 157 candles to blow out. Mel and Emily had designed the cake. On top of the cake was a marzipan sculpture of a cow's head, and below the cow a plaque that read, 'To the biggest cow in Colorado.'

It was wonderful to be sung to by a crew full of great-looking men. Even so, I took a sleeping pill that night so I didn't have to think about how many birthdays I have left.

20 April 2022

We were in Aspen, the swankiest ski resort of them all. Aspen started out as a poor mining town where people came to find gold. The mines dried up and people stopped coming, and then someone with a brain thought, 'I know, let's turn it into a ski resort and charge $800 for a ski pass.'

It's now Beverly Hills on a slope where the streets are lined, not in gold, but with Prada, Gucci, Valentino, Chanel, Dior, all so handy for purchasing ski wear. And God bless 'em, they have for sale ski clothes lined in the fur of animals that are nearly extinct, handbags made out of the chins of antelope (the softest part and the most expensive), polar bear hats and boots with diamonds on the heels. The idea is to bring in a sugar daddy, point at something expensive, and then he buys.

Our guide had been a professional snowboarder when she was young, but after she became a drug addict and was thrown into jail a few times, her career ended. She told us that a few years later, miraculously she got a job modelling and became a mini celeb by doing ads for suntan lotion. She was able to crawl her way back up to being a pro again. She showed us a photo of herself in Alaska. She was coming down a sheer cliff on a snowboard. Unfortunately en route she broke every bone in her body. Everyone has a story.

Our guide mentioned casually that Aspen had the wildest, richest party people in America, as well as a high rate of suicide. I thought that was an odd thing to tell us. In the afternoon she took us to a shop on the main street called Kimo Sabe. This is where the uber-wealthy come to buy cowboy hats that start at £6,000. She told us Jeff Bezos went into space wearing one of their hats. Like I'm going to buy a hat immediately with that information.

The shop was filled with American Indian costumes made of mink and gems and the walls were lined with cowboy hats waiting for some sucker to try one on. The minute you do, you're mobbed by bushy-tailed salesgirls gabbling at 700 miles per minute, serving you champagne and getting you so hyped up that they can convince you to buy accessories, which drives up the price of the hat. Diamond hat bands cost an extra £10,000, feathers cost £2,000, silver pins cost £3,000 each. It keeps going up until your hat doesn't look like a hat, it's a giant pile of bling. Some hats are so weighed down, you try it on, you break your neck. If you're a 'big spender' you're invited 'upstairs' to the private club where you can get anything, I mean anything for the right price. The girls were humping the air on top of the bar, blaring into a bullhorn to inform us it was drinks time, 'Come and get it studs n' gals.' (It's always drinks time.) And you chug the most expensive things that have ever been chugged. Some drinks had gold poured into them. I thought when it comes back out of me, I'm going straight to a pawnbroker. The girls yanked the three of us up on top of the bar to dance with them. I went rigid with mortification. I was next to Emily, who knew how to move in a 'lap-dancery' kind of way. The bar girls tried to give me confidence telling me how hot I looked. But I have seen the rushes and I was the opposite of hot. I contemplated offering money to the production to not show that particular dance number, but I knew it would be futile. We all left the store with hats worth the cost of my mortgage.

21 April 2022

We drove up the Moab Mountains, which are made out of gigantic red boulders that look like sculptures you'd expect to find on the moon. My driver told me she travels around the country 365 days a year in her open-top jeep. She said she's following her dream by never stopping. She had put a cage on top of the car; that way, if the jeep flipped over, she'd just hang upside down from her seatbelt and wait until someone came along to cut her out. I asked where she slept, since there was no roof, and she said she loves to sleep in nature: rain or snow or hurricane. Sometimes in fifteen below zero she'd build a fire in a hole, throw over a tarp and sleep on it. I had found another modern-day Isabella. Driven, never standing still, and perhaps running away from something. Who knows?

I would have interviewed her for the film, but during the conversation we were driving vertically up a rock and I had to vomit. When I got out at the top, the wind must have been going forty miles an hour. I told the camera crew to stand back and duck because I didn't want what came out of me to blow on to them. (How's that for courtesy?) Luckily, I have a strong pelvic floor and was able to hold it down.

At the end of the day, they took us to some 'hee-haw' cowboy Victorian town. The hotel we walked into could have been a brothel; maroon velvet decor and fringes lining everything. There was a bluegrass band, and we were invited to sing along. Mel refused, though she would have blown the bluegrass band off the planet if they'd figured out who she was. She didn't want to make a fool of herself, I guess, but I had pretty much only made a fool of myself from the start, so I sang a selection of my old camp songs. After a while, people got upset because I never found the right key due to being tone deaf. Not my fault.

24 April 2022

Today we went to a sanctuary for wolves that've had a bad experience out in the wild, which in my opinion is exactly where they belong. They're much bigger in person than they are in photos. We were put in a pen with them, and told to stay still because they're 'friendly'. So friendly, I was licked by several of them while shitting myself. We got a lecture from the woman in charge, who informed us that wolves are misunderstood. They will only attack you if you attack first.

While I was being licked by one wolf, another had pulled my copy of the Isabella book out of my back pocket and was trying to eat it. The woman told the 'friendly' wolf calmly to give her the book. He growled, baring his fangs, until she gave up. I thought he was going to tear her arm off. When he finally got tired of chewing the book, he dropped it. My whole raison d'être for doing the documentary was now covered in saliva and ripped to shreds.

27 April 2022

When they told us that today we'd be going to search for Sasquatch, I thought they meant a vegetable. It turned out they meant Bigfoot, the legendary monster who supposedly roams the backwoods. We were introduced to a woman who claimed to have had several sightings of Bigfoot. She recalled with shaky voice and spooked eyes how one night she heard grunting noises, and when she came out of the house, there it was standing in front of her car. She knew who it was because it was eight feet tall and covered in hair, and guess what? It had big feet. She was a member of the police force, so clearly her descriptions are on the ball and accurate.

What's more unnerving is that she still works for the police department. In my opinion, these are the type of folks who claim to have been abducted, brought on to a UFO and forced to have sexual encounters with a Third Kind.

That evening there was a campfire where a Bigfoot expert showed us unequivocal proof of its existence: photos of scratch marks on a tent, paw prints on a tree trunk, long hairs left on a fern. Bigfoot was last seen in these parts, so after hours of endless stories we went into the forest with our infrared goggles. Then Emily claimed something, probably Bigfoot, had touched her. (Why wouldn't he? She's gorgeous.) Emily became hysterical and was carried off sobbing to a tent.

I turned around to face the camera, intending to sum up the show. I was going to say that when people first came to America to dig for gold, they had boundless hope in their hearts because they believed in life, liberty and the pursuit of happiness. They didn't realize until many years later that gold wouldn't buy them happiness. That's what I was planning to say. But when I looked around, the camera crew had disappeared. They were in the tent consoling Emily.

30 April 2022

This was the last day of the shoot, when the three of us would have to climb up Pikes Peak. When Isabella climbed Pikes Peak, she wore a Hawaiian dress and shoes three sizes too big. I don't know what Mountain Jim was wearing. In the scene we're dressed in 2-foot thick down jackets, five pairs of socks and thermals up the wazoo. Emily was complaining her ass was frozen because she was wearing a thong. A climbing thong? Soon after we started our ascent, the winds picked up to 50 mph. We couldn't even see each other, but what's worse, our makeup was running down our faces.

We had almost reached the summit when Emily fell between two rocks, twisting her ankle. She started crying from the pain. I wondered if I should drag her up by the arms and hair. Wasn't that what Mountain Jim did when Isabella was slipping, and almost fainted? I was trying to read from the book to find out exactly what Jim did to save her, but the book was too stained with wolf saliva and my tears were blinding me. I ended up dragging Emily to the summit, and as night fell and with the winds lashing ice into our eyes, we finished this story of three women in show business, bucking up their careers. Needless to say the three of us bonded through adversity and comedy. I shouldn't have done this crammed between two of my journeys for the book.

6

Christianity

When we are lazy, we stay on the path we are already on, even if it is going nowhere. Everything winds down unless some outside force winds it back up.

– M. Scott Peck, *The Road Less Travelled*

When I came back, Ed asked me what the filming had been like, and I started to babble. Not words. Just babble. He looked concerned.

With my hands shaking, I showed him photos of the most stunning ice-covered peaks of the Rockies, and he said, 'It looks beautiful. What was the problem, Ruby?'

I answered, 'I climbed them.'

I'd had no preparation. The words, 'You're going to climb 15,000 feet' were not mentioned anywhere. I did not want to be shown up by Mel or Emily again, so I practically skipped up that mountain with the high ice winds blasting off my facial features so that icicles hung from my nose. When the cameras were turned off, every muscle I've ever owned went into spasm but God damn it I got to the top before Mel and Emily. Isabella would have been proud of me.

As I look back, again the timing of everything was destined for disaster. I had climbed 15,000 feet and now a mere three days later, I was going to visit a Christian monastery. Ed said, hopelessly, 'Ruby, why don't you slow down?' There was no reply expected.

If I'd had a few more days before the visit to recuperate, I might have been fine, but when I took the train to Leeds, I was exhausted and losing my marbles. Not so much a mission to find meaning any more, now it was a mission of madness.

Why did I choose this particular monastery in the first place? The idea was inspired by an interview I did with *The Times* about my book *And Now for the Good News*. Richard Coles began the interview by saying that thirty years earlier he had seen my magnificent performance as a whore/nun in *Measure for Measure* at the Royal Shakespeare Company.

In this production, Juliet Stevenson and I had been cast in non-speaking roles but managed to upstage most of the actors who had lines. While they did their Shakespearean couplets we were standing around in slut-uesque poses. Both of us had covered ourselves not just in pox marks but buboes we made out of rubber. (Buboes, for those of you not in the know, were pus-filled boils that were symptoms of the plague.)

The Black Death was rife in seventeenth-century London, and our whores were obviously on their last legs, gasping for air but still open for business. No one could tear their eyes away from Juliet and me as we over-acted with no lines. Clearly Richard couldn't, because thirty years later here he was telling me he still remembered my sensational non-speaking role as a whore/nun. (Juliet wasn't as good as I was. He didn't remember her.)

When I told Richard about the book of journeys I was writing, he suggested I visit the Christian monastery where he had trained to become a vicar. I joked I might become a nun. In the article he wrote later, Richard mentioned that he'd seen me at the start of my career playing a nun and he would see me out as a nun.

Richard offered to speak to the Brethren, and he said that if they agreed to a visit, he could escort me there and stay a few days. When he called me back with the date I should have delayed; I mean, the Christian monastery wasn't going anywhere. I said, 'Book me!'

It made sense to include religious faith in my book but I had only given myself a week to investigate, so I stuck with learning everything I could about Jews and Christians. I love all their rituals: how everyone does the same thing at the same time all together. (See Thanksgiving, but don't eat a turkey.) I loved almost everything I was investigating, except I couldn't go along with the God bit. The problem is I don't believe in anything. Non-belief can be seen as a sign of a liberated mind, but it means living in no man's land. There's no one to light a candle with or join in a Gregorian chant at Michaelmas time.

I grew up with Jewish traditions but I don't know much about them. I do know there's one where you get money for finding the hidden matzo (it's always about money for my people) and eat food that symbolizes things, like horseradish which reminds them how bitter they were about something that happened thousands of years ago. (Like they need reminding? I know no Jew who isn't bitter – mainly me.)

I never embraced the religion I was born into. When I was ten, I was kicked out of Sunday School class. I had to stand in the hallway. I was flicking a light switch on and off to entertain myself when the Rabbi flew up to me, robes flapping behind him. He dragged me into the synagogue and pointed to the eternal light. It was off! I had turned off the eternal light! Because I committed that felony, I was asked to leave. And that's when Judaism and I parted ways. But I thought I'd better give Judaism one last whirl, so I met up with a wonderful Rabbi. I'll call him RG. He agreed to answer some of the myriad questions that were bothering me, like if the Ten Commandments were so important, how come when Moses dropped them, he didn't get into trouble? RG was a very patient man.

R: *So I'm Jewish but it has never captured me. I like the food they serve on Friday night but that's about it. I would love to have rituals in my life, to celebrate supposed holy days but I just don't believe in anything. When the Jews ask, 'Why would this night be different from other nights?' I have no idea.*

RG: *What's different from a Friday night dinner to a Thursday or Monday night dinner? Jewish tradition is based on ritual. Friday night dinner is a time to be with family and friends and the shared ritual means everyone has a common ground, no matter how much they argue in the week. It begins by making three blessings, to the candles, wine, and bread.*

R: *Very Christian sounding so far.*

RG: *Okay, so let's start with the candles. When they're lit, Friday night begins. You could say the candles are an ancient technology, to acknowledge the Sabbath or the Jewish day of rest. It happens each week from sunset on Friday to sunset on Saturday. For the next twenty-four hours they aren't going to do anything, not work, not exercise, not even turn on or off lights, not use technology.*

R: *That's me out.*

RG: *Then after twenty-four hours, another candle is lit to mark the end of the Sabbath. The idea of Shabbat is that God made the world in six days and on the seventh rested, so we do the same.*

R: *What a great excuse. I'm going to use that. I'm putting that on my answer machine: 'Hello – I'm Jewish, I can't answer the phone right now, don't leave a message until I light another candle.' Where did Jews get the idea God made the world in six days?*

RG: *The Bible isn't meant to be read as a literal text. It's an allegorical text. So when the Bible says God created the world in six days, we now know six days can be 6 billion years. But the idea was that there was an intentional creation of this world. God wanted a world that was ordered, and created us to morally interpret that world.*

R: *So you believe man is basically good?*

RG: *I think we're created to wrestle with what it means to be good. If I rated humanity, I would say we are failing in what God wants us to do.*

R: *If there is a God he must be so disappointed.*

RG: *We don't know if we're here by accident or on purpose. I'm going to choose 'on purpose', because I would like to know that my life is not just an accident. The created world that we live in is not succeeding. Nature's being messed up. I'm not saying that individuals don't make good choices, but humanity as a whole has made bad choices.*

R: *So where do you get your sense of meaning?*

RG: *If I woke up every morning thinking the next twenty-four hours were about me and only me, it would be less meaningful*

*than believing that there is greater purpose and greater con-
nectivity in this world than just me and my life. I need to
understand myself as having a purpose greater than just my
biology.*

R: *So you believe it's God that makes you have purpose?*

RG: *Well, what is greater than yourself? You don't have to call it
God. Call it Bob or Molly. It's the thing that I think all religions
are trying to connect us to. To make us feel we're part of something bigger.*

R: *I think the ideal purpose is being of service. I know already when
I do something for no other reason than it helps someone, I feel
better.*

RG: *Yes, it's that, but prayer also gives purpose.*

R: *I don't know how to do that.*

RG: *You told me that you do your forty-five minutes of mindfulness
a day. I would say that's your prayer. The word for prayer in Heb-
rew is to 'fill up'. And that word grammatically comes from the
root 'to judge'. It means reflexive judging. So prayer, to me, is a
constant self-checking. When you're meditating, sitting for forty-
five minutes, even if forty-four of those minutes were meaningless,
in that one minute if you become more peaceful and that affects
people around you for the better, that's being of service. That's
what good religion does. Good religion creates communities that
experience peace together. So on Friday night Shabbat, it's a spiritual practice to allow people to let go of the week, have moments
of reflection and then spread it out to others.*

R: *I love the community part but I'd be a hypocrite if I said I
could show up in a synagogue and feel part of it. I can't but*

I wish I could. It's too bad because I'd like my daughters to marry Jewish men for shallow reasons, not religious . . . But that's beside the point.

*

So, when Richard invited me to visit his Christian community, I thought why not try it? Who knows, miracles happen, and maybe someone there could convert me.

Richard had phoned to tell me he couldn't be there for the first few days, so I took the train to Leeds alone and unescorted to visit the Brothers in Christ at Mirfield at the Community of the Resurrection.

7 May 2022

My first impression of the buildings of the Community of the Resurrection was that they were very austere: grey stone, dark windows, very early Victorian. But though they were dark on the outside, there was light within. On entering I was greeted by a very loving, 'the-mother-I-wish-I-had' type. I can't resist those. She led me to my room, which was fifteen feet by eight feet, similar to the one at Spirit Rock. There were no closets or drawers, a single bed and a tiny sink. It looked more like a cell than a room, but it was exactly the kind of place where I can feel safe. From the bed I could see the doorknob turn if someone was going to burst in.

After the woman closed the door behind her, I dropped into bed and curled up into a ball. I knew it would take great effort to lift myself up again but I'd been invited to have dinner with the Brethren. I knew being a no-show would be incredibly rude. When the time came, I dragged myself out of bed and I went to meet the Brothers for the first time.

They were charming, smart, and completely got my sense of humour. I told them I had a problem believing in Jesus. They said they sometimes had a problem believing too but what kept them going was their faith. How do you have faith but not believe in the product?

When I looked into their eyes, what I saw reflected back was non-judgemental love. Something else to be jealous of. Why can't I just make the jump and take the plunge into those Baptism waters?

I asked what kind of Christians they were. They told me they follow the gospel life as recorded in the Acts of the Apostles. They're rooted in the Anglican tradition and formed in a Benedictine round of worship. I understood nothing about what they were saying. I felt like I was a visitor from another planet.

I was introduced to the head of the community. In a movie, he would have been cast as the priest who has the ear of the Pope. He was dignified and charismatic. Let's call him B.

R: *I wish I could join the flock but I just can't. Here's the problem I have and you can tell me to leave. I really can't go along with the idea that Jesus was the son of God. I'm sure Jesus was enchanting and no doubt he was a great influencer but the God being his father thing is way out of my realm.*

B: *I think for me just believing in Jesus doesn't quite cut it. And I don't think one suddenly becomes a Christian. You've got to work at it. It's a daily effort. And sometimes I don't want to do it.*

R: *So what makes it worth doing?*

B: It's worth it because I have things to do at certain times, the boundaries are clear, and that frees up your mind to be able to think clearly about things. It's liberating.

R: With nothing to think about except getting to the church on time, I'm sure your mind is completely de-cluttered. I'm so jealous.

B: Well, you're not just getting up at 5.00am for yourself. You're getting up for your brothers and sisters, too. And they make it easier. If I wasn't living here, I'd find it difficult to keep up a personal prayer life because I'm kind of a lazy person. But there's something about the daily routines of morning prayer and evening prayer that keep me going. It also helps that I meditate. When my mind strays, I take my focus back to the Gospel.

R: That's exactly how I use mindfulness except I don't focus back on the Gospel bit. Obviously. I focus on my breath.

B: As I see it, to practise mindfulness is to show compassion for oneself. It is a good act. And we believe when someone performs a good act for themselves or others, Jesus is behind it.

R: You can't be good without Jesus in the picture?

B: We believe that any goodness in this world comes from the Spirit of God.

R: So that's the only way you can do good? If he's involved?

B: God isn't only there when you're doing good. One of the times I felt closest to God was when my mother died. It was terrible. But God felt utterly, utterly close.

R: In that situation I would 'Rage, rage against the dying of the light.'

I was showing off how educated I was so he'd think I was smart, but then he quoted the whole Dylan Thomas poem at me and that put me in my place.

I told B I had to go and do a Zoom call. I wanted to give him the idea that okay, maybe I wasn't so smart but I was terribly important. I didn't have a Zoom call. I wanted to go to bed, so I lied to him. I lied to a priest. I think he probably knew I didn't have a Zoom call, but he still looked at me with non-judgemental love. These guys just won't stop giving.

When I got to my room, I locked the door and collapsed on the bed. The bed is usually my happy place but something felt wrong. At first I thought maybe I had a virus, or jet-lag. Then I remembered feeling the same way years ago but I couldn't put my finger on what it was, until a sudden lightning flash hit me. Could it be depression rearing its head again? After a twelve-year absence, could that old evil chestnut have come back?

To me, depression is like being possessed. You would think at a Christian monastery, Satan wouldn't have the nerve to show up. I wondered if I should ask the head of the Brethren to give me an exorcism. But it might be rude to take up so much of his time when I was supposed to be a guest.

I called my psychiatrist to tell him I was spiralling downhill. He said he could hear by the sound of my voice that I was in trouble, and that I should come back to London. When he said that, I felt that shame we depressives usually feel at some point, like I was being self-indulgent, making the whole thing up for attention and I should just shut up.

After the call, I missed dinner and slept sixteen hours. In one of my dreams, Isabella Bird was suing me for not giving her enough airtime. I woke up tired. Darkness was descending fast.

8 May 2022

I ran through the hallways. The first service of the day was at 7.30am. It was to be followed by a 12.00am, 3.00pm, 6.00pm and 9.00pm service. I couldn't tell if it was early or late but I knew to run. Time loses all meaning when you're ill. But sick or not, I was going to go to all of the services and get me some 'faith'.

Space loses meaning too in my condition. The hallways turned into a maze. I was lost. Everywhere I went there seemed to be the same paintings of Mary and her son. I was going to be very, very late. I started to panic.

I found the hushed echoey church, but the service had started and I had to find a pew. You could hear my shoes clip-clopping across the stones like I was on loudspeakers.

The church was designed minimally: white walls, a simple white altar and not much Jesusy decoration. When someone hit the organ, the Brethren entered in procession in black outfits. The two in the front carried long candlesticks with lit candles at the end, the last two were swinging the incense.

A kind lady handed me a hymn sheet. She could have been the same one who let me in; they all looked 'Mrs Doubtfire' to me. The lyrics said something about how when we die Jesus will lifteth us up. That even the cows and whales should bless him. He would even lifteth up the very old who make it to seventy. I was startled to hear that because I'm heading in the same direction and I thought Jesus probably knows how old I am.

A priestess got up and walked to the altar. She was very

articulate. She told us that although the Jews were throwing stones at Jesus, he still forgiveth them. I was slightly alarmed, thinking I might have been related to one of those stoners, and hoping the Brethren wouldn't find out.

I wanted so badly to feel the spirit enter into me, to be able to rise to my feet, speaking in tongues, frothing and shouting, 'Hallelujah!' Everyone sang again. Psalm 409. They're so random, those numbers! I thought I was singing along as well until I put my finger in my ear to hear my voice. I discovered I was singing gobbledegook and that key-wise I was on Jupiter.

9 May 2022

Next morning I had breakfast with B. I pretended everything was normal. Over our cornflakes, we continued the interview.

R: *What did you do before you were a priest?*

B: *My background was politics. I was a local council candidate, involved in campaigning. I was always passionate about making people's lives better and to make the world a better place. But I slowly realized that actually with politics, you're always expecting something in return.*

R: *Like doing good to get more votes?*

B: *Yes, exactly, it was too much about what I wanted. I quit politics. I got a calling and I came here where there's no hidden agenda. In church it's not about what we want, it's about what God wants. There's a selflessness to it. When we're in church and we're praying, we want to hear God, we want God to speak* to us, otherwise what's the point? And it's not about getting something in an instant. God's playing the long game. We have to not expect the votes. Life's about slogging on. Getting on with it.

*

That night Richard showed up. Richard is charming and has wit coming out of his ears. He gave me a tour of the ecclesiastical school where he became a vicar after being in the Communards – a 1980s pop duo. He showed me an ancient amphitheatre where they put on *A Chorus Line* when he was a student there. He played The Chorus. The mind boggles. The rest of the clergy in fishnets. He goes into my top ten list of the campest people I've ever met. I told him I had a Zoom call and ran back to my bed.

10 May 2022

When I got up I knew full well I had depression. It's like finally admitting you have pneumonia because the X-rays show it, that's how clearly I knew I had it. There can be no doubt. Once you're in it, you hardly know where you are. You don't exist any more. Your spirit has left the building. Your body is no longer connected to your mind and you can't figure out who's moving your limbs.

I knew I wouldn't be able to fake it any more. I knocked on Richard's door. I told him I had to leave the monastery, that I was very ill, and I wasn't being a wanker – he probably thought I was anyway – and I was sorry. So sorry, so very sorry!

My psychiatrist called to tell me he had booked me into a

clinic and that I should get to London and check in. Richard drove me to the train station. I was pretending I was still Ruby but I didn't have a clue how she used to act. I tried hard to be light and amusing but it was just snippets of sentences that fell out of my mouth. I was a poor imitation of myself.

After Richard dropped me off at the train station, I started experiencing familiar sensations from the past as clearly as if it was yesterday. The hands on the station clock were jumping around staccato fashion. I recognized the feeling of not being able to tell a minute from an hour. I needed to get somewhere safe.

I walked into a too-loud café and stood like a Zombie unable to decide whether I should ask for a cup of tea, or go outside and throw myself in front of the train. The mental torment was mounting fast.

I missed a few trains because I wasn't sure how long the train doors were kept open, and I was frightened I'd be half in, half out when the door closed and I'd get dragged down the line.

When I got to London, it took a long time to get off the train because I was too scared the doors would shut on me. I had written the name of the clinic on a crumpled-up piece of paper, handed it to the taxi driver and off I went on my latest adventure. Not a journey to find meaning, but a journey towards a fully-fledged breakdown.

11 May 2022

They were expecting me, so I was met at the door. Someone led me upstairs to a room that was a dead-body beige. They had removed anything you could use to hang yourself from. A nurse handed me forms to fill in. They asked questions like was I suicidal, did I feel I wanted to kill someone, and how old I was. I filled in everything but lied about my age. I'm not that crazy.

Other nurses came and went. I was given some pills to swallow. The pills made my brain fall into warm water, like it had been on fire.

I didn't come out of my room for I don't know how many days. I never opened the curtains. I needed darkness to match mine. I hunkered down because there was a typhoon of mental torture raging inside.

7

Back to the Clinic

9 June 2022

Bang bang bang I'm under the rTMS for my twentieth session; my last one. I hadn't noticed much of a change from these treatments, but now, at the last treatment, I can see a very small chink of light. It takes as long to notice depression coming and going as it does watching your hair grow. What's different today is rather than give the technician grief, I thanked him. When I first clapped eyes on him, I thought he was an unemployed person who had snuck in off the street, stolen a plastic apron and was pretending to be a neuroscientist. I used to quiz him before the sessions started about where he went to school? Did he in fact go to school? How old was he exactly? (He looked fourteen.) He'd tell me he was trained by an expert in rTMS procedures, and I'd wonder, 'Why did I get the trainee? Why didn't I get the expert?' I used to grill him on how a magnetic hammer slamming the right side of my head could possibly be healing me. Today I'm not grilling him because I have to admit it's beginning to work. When I was last admitted to a mental clinic for chronic depression, twelve years ago, it took me five months to recover; this time it's been five weeks and the veil of doom seems to be lifting. Maybe he's not a liar after all. He told me at the beginning there was a 60% success rate from rTMS in the clinic. At the time, I didn't believe him, but this could be the reason I'm no longer in the 'walking dead' camp. I don't feel like hurling myself at a moving car any more. Now, when I'm crossing the road, I look both ways. I have no intention of ending my days as roadkill.

I can tell things are shifting. Five weeks ago I couldn't have conceived I'd be walking downstairs to the scheduled therapy classes or the cafeteria. (The elevator is still broken.) Now I bolt down, rushing past fellow inmates who are in the state I used to be in. They're clutching the handrail for dear life, afraid they may float away into thin air if they let go. Some of the inmates haven't changed much since I've been here. They're still sitting glassy-eyed in the corridor; still looking lost. The lights have gone out. When I try to listen to their stories, they just repeat the mantra of all people suffering with a mental illness, which is, 'Will this ever end?'

I'm getting a fondness for the place. I hated it at first, but I've started to feel at home here. I even like my room: the no-view window, the hanger-less closets, the faucet-less shower, the suitcase that I live out of, and the books that I've never read.

10 June 2022

My son Max comes to visit me. He takes me to a new and even more kitsch coffee place he's researched. Max has hit a bull's-eye. This one is a Mexican coffee shop. The waitresses sing traditional songs alongside a recording of sombreroed trumpeters blaring so loud it will blow your facial hair off. Even though it's only a recording it still sounds like a herd of elephants charging at you. The customers have to join in for the 'Olé'. The servers don't seem to understand much English and they get our orders wrong. I got choritos instead of cappuccino, which is an easy mistake to make. Max looks at me with nervous eyes as if this is going to throw me back into the darkness, but when he sees I'm laughing, you can feel his relief.

On our way back to the clinic we pass a church. There's a sign outside. It says there's a candlelight concert that night. I want to go. Max tries to get tickets but they're sold out.

Later that night, I go back to the church. (This is a woman too afraid to cross her room a few weeks ago.) They're still sold out, so I do what I've done for most of my life, I jump the queue. When I get to the door, I tell the ticket taker that the friend I'm with has my ticket but she's inside. She doesn't believe me and tells me to get lost. (Another of the million people who don't recognize me.) The two women behind me interrupt. They say they have an extra ticket, and give it to me. As we take our seats in the balcony, I look down: there seem to be a thousand lit candles surrounding the stage. The scene is breathtakingly eerie. There is a grand piano in the middle of the stage. Enter a ravishing Asian female violinist and a pianist in a tuxedo. They begin playing Mozart amid the flickering glow. So there I am in rapture, listening and thinking, 'Why did I never do this before?' This music goes straight into my heart and I start to experience emotions I haven't felt for a long time. At the interval, I talk to the two women. They tell me that they live together in the East End, and they're getting married soon. I can tell, they're very much in love. Then they ask where I live, and I tell them I'm living in a mental ward. One of the women says she guessed something was wrong with me. I ask how she knew and she says it's because my phone keeps beeping with texts saying, 'Are you okay?' I hadn't noticed.

After the performance ends, the women walk me back to the clinic. As we say goodnight to each other, they invite me to come for tea at their house any time I feel like it. I think how kind the world can be sometimes and I walk into the building where I will get my meds to go to sleep. I'm loving it here.

11 June 2022

I've fallen in love with a Jamaican nurse called Risk. I greet her daily with, 'Hi Risk.' Even though it's probably my worst joke ever, I think I'm getting my sense of humour back. I'm sure she's heard that joke a thousand times, but Risk laughs with such joy, it's infectious.

Whenever she visits my room, she booms, 'Give me a hug, Ruby!' Then she cocoons me in such strong maternal arms that I want to live there forever.

After we finish hugging, she tells me to pick three affirmation cards. She fans out a deck she carries around in her pocket. If anyone other than Risk offered me an affirmation card, I'd roll my eyes, but I'll go along with anything she says. So I take a random card.

The first affirmation card reads, 'It's during our darkest moments that we must focus on the light.' A quote from Aristotle Onassis. I wouldn't have thought Onassis had a dark moment, floating around in his King Kong-sized yacht with Jackie O in the kitchen. But clearly he did, otherwise why would he have wasted his time writing it?

The second card reads, 'We suffer more often in imagination than in reality.' This was a quote from Seneca. I don't believe mental illness is a result of the imagination, so Seneca will be eliminated from my Christmas card list from now on. The third and last card was a good one, though.

'You've become so damaged that when someone tries to give you what you deserve, you either sabotage it or you push them away because you don't know what to do with it.' The author wasn't identified, but I bet he/she is somewhere in this clinic.

12 June 2022

Shrink session

The shrink has a glow around her today – like a lightbulb went on inside of her.

R: *I must be getting better because I can see that my life before wasn't as bad as I imagined.*

S: *You start to recover your memory once you're getting well again. Depression dampens down the memory because your mind is using most of its energy to try and make sense of the distorted thinking.*

R: *I've felt safe here even though it's a mental ward version of* Fawlty Towers. *I feel so close to everyone here. I've got a new community. Some people want a husband. Some people want a threesome. I want at least twenty people around me and no sex.*

S: *Because you've always had this fear of being pulled back into your parents' house, you honed the skill of being able to form a group around you. It's your way of protecting yourself. You didn't have a connection in your home. There's no image of a mother, there's no image of a father. Aloneness for you is dangerous. You also developed the ability to get deep with people quite quickly.*

R: *Sometimes I just need bodies, it doesn't matter if I know them or not.*

S: *There's nothing wrong with needing people as long as you're aware that when you're drawn towards protective groups of women to soothe you, it's because you have trouble soothing yourself. But there is something more contemplative about you now. A few months ago, you weren't able to go into your house in London without being highly activated into a very distressed, very dysregulated state. You're learning to observe yourself rather than just react to circumstances. You're aware of what creates chaos in you and what gives you balance.*

R: *I'm sometimes scared that if I know too much about myself I'll lose my edge or I'll become too self-conscious.*

S: *You're not suddenly going to lose that highly driven part of you. That's what allowed you to deal with your trauma, your ability to be funny and be incisive. But it also came with desperation. You're much more able to talk to me now. You were pretty angry before, whereas now you seem to have become more reflective.*

R: *Yeah. Well, I was angry. My anger was driving everything.*

S: *You've come so far.*

R: *Can I say something funny now?*

S: *No.*

*

I don't know why I never noticed this thing called trauma before but when everyone loves you, you never have to dig deep. Only when the attention starts to dim and people lose their interest in you, do you get that nudge from your intuition that something isn't right, that there's a monster, let's call it trauma, lurking down below. Sometimes I wish the shrink had let it sleep but she wouldn't stop drilling away. (Can you believe I paid for that?) My trauma was like that alien they pulled out of John Hurt's stomach in the film. (See how far I've come, Oprah?)

Before she went off Zoom the shrink said she would email me a copy of a story that would resonate with me. This is it. It's called 'The Good Fairy'.

From the corners where the silence remains, there came the urgency to go to a mountain top and scream out the whole truth.

Rose sent out a prayer to God, to the universe: 'It's too painful, I can't take it!' Then she came to Rose, the power of mind, the energy of the universe, the Good Fairy in The Wizard of Oz, *waving a wand.*

Rose sat cross-legged on the floor of her bedroom, looking up; she was about eight years old. The Good Fairy said, 'Here's the deal. There's just too much going on here and I don't have the power to make it be gone, to make it be okay, or even to help you cope with it in a way that's not going to cause you some pain.

'What I can do,' said the Good Fairy, 'is help you get through this time now, help you get through it as it is going on. It will come back, but it will come back to you only at a later time, when you're able to handle it and there will be someone to help you.' Rose said, 'Okay, because I can't take it any more.'

The Good Fairy waved her wand, saying: 'I am going to send the painful things that are happening into different parts of your body, and your body will hold them for you like it's a time capsule.

'Your heart, your heart is broken and I'm going to have to let your rib cage close in around it and let your heart constrict so that you don't feel the pain of your heart breaking.

'I'm going to really need to tighten up your neck to let it be a fortress with very thick round walls, so that what you are feeling doesn't get up to your mouth, and you can't speak the words. You can't cry out for help and can't scream out in rage. You won't be able to breathe too deeply, to feel what's going on in your body. That fortress will keep the knowledge of what's happening in your body from connecting with your head, so that you will not be fully conscious of what's going on.

'I will tie up your ears, so that you hear but you won't take too much in. And this is what I will do with your mind. It will store the truth in a deep, deep place, sealed away behind steel doors of fear. This will for now help you to live with, accept and believe the lies you are told. The lie that you deserve this and that this is the way your life has to be.

'When the time is right, you will begin to open up. It will be a very long process. It may take as long to heal as you've been in pain and in the frozen place. Finally, your body will no longer be able to hold all this in. Your muscles will begin to give way, you will feel an urgency to do physical healing, and that will begin the process of really unwinding your body and releasing everything you've been holding all these years. There will be physical as well as emotional pain in the process.

'By then you will be strong enough, safe enough and old enough to bear the truth and you will have a special friend, who will be the grown-up – adult – you, your Self, who will hold you as no one else can, as you find yourself again.

'Now I want you to go to bed. I will wave my wand and you will go to sleep, and when you wake up, you will forget

I was ever here. You will forget you asked for help and you will no longer feel your daily pain. This is the only way I know to get you through this.'

I don't know what it is with that shrink. Sometimes I feel she's too sappy for words but she means well.

13 June 2022

My curiosity is back. I don't want to stay in my room any more. I want to find out why everyone's here: what's their prognosis? I've begun taking regular visits to the cafeteria. It wasn't easy to find at first because this place is all winding hallways and ramps. Once I get a tray, I pick out something edible or at least something I think I recognize by its colour or shape. After I pick out who looks craziest in the café, I make a beeline for the seat next to them. Today it was an elderly woman in a stained nightgown with high velvet go-go boots. She's in full makeup, though her red lipstick is nowhere near her lips, and she wears a silver crown made out of foil. She informs me there was shrimp in her freezer but wolves came to her house and stole the frozen shrimp, so she started leaving vegan moussaka out, which didn't stop the wolves stealing her shrimp, because they didn't care for her vegan moussaka. I tell her I'm fascinated that she thought the wolves were vegan. She looks at me like I'm crazy as if to say, 'It's obvious they're vegan, you idiot.'

The rest of the table are cutters. I ask to see some of their wounds, which they proudly show me. The ones who come across jolliest have the deepest wounds. I compliment them when I see a particularly imaginative design. That makes them smile.

I started practising mindfulness again a few days ago. I stopped when I came to the clinic, because when you're in the depths of depression there's no sense in doing it because you haven't got a mind. Now I'm toughening up my mental muscles again to be able to cool my brain down before it goes on a rampage like it did weeks ago.

People, including those with mental problems, deserve respect, and that is something some of the nurses here need to learn. Some nurses are sensational, like Risk, some don't even look at you when you speak to them. You can tell who the newby depressives are. They're the ones who only repeat that one question: 'Will this ever end?' I'm able to tell them with confidence that I got better and I promise if they hold on, they will too. A few bi-polars are talking a million miles per minute, deliriously happy to be here and very busy even though there's not much to do. There are a few Americans who believe they're running a nail salon, because they give each other pedicures all day long while they're chattering like wild hyenas on amphetamine. The best activity of all happens in the garden. Even when it's freezing outside, God bless them, the smokers are in their corner lighting up. If you can get down there I would recommend it. They will give you the finest of stories – far better than at any show in the West End – and if you're in need of a light or a cigarette, they will happily oblige.

14 June 2022

During the evenings, I've been getting antsy, so I started booking other candlelight concerts. At the start, I still had my old habit of booking for sometimes two concerts in one evening, all on at the same time. Still addicted to that old adrenaline rush by being late for both events. A double shot of panic. I'd run between the chamber music orchestra in St James's Church and a piano recital in St Martin in the Fields, Trafalgar Square. I was running most of the time, so I missed a lot of both concerts.

Tonight – this is a big step for me – I'm only going to one concert. I arrived early and I didn't have the lonely feeling I used to get if I walked into an event on my own. I was watching a brilliant pianist, whose fingers were moving so fast they were a blur, like a hummingbird, but landed like feathers on the keys. The pianist was a beautiful young girl in an off-the-shoulder black satin evening dress. She was curled over in concentration, her neck long, and blonde hair had started falling out from its elegant French roll. I could feel a pinch of the usual 'I want to be her' envy starting to simmer, but I held it in check. I thought who wants to practise scales most of your life? Not me. She probably doesn't have much of a life anyway. I left glad I wasn't her, even though I would have loved that neck.

15 June 2022

I go out with my family and two friends to a Chinese restaurant called Royal China. We find out from the waiter there's a Royal China private club next door. I have to know what the difference is between the club and the restaurant with the same name. My curiosity is clearly making a comeback. I stroll into the club like I'm a member. My kids and my girlfriend are bringing up the rear. I discover the club is exactly the same as the restaurant we were just in, with one slight difference. There are security guards to ensure non-members don't get in. The moment I enter illegally, I am manhandled by security. I start fighting them off, insisting I am meeting a friend. My girlfriend who came in with me cleverly says, 'Oh, there she is,' and she points into a private room. I struggle out of their grip and run into the room where she is pointing. There I see a masterpiece of cosmetic surgery; this woman has had so much work done she looks like a blowfish. Her eyes are stretched like slits in a forest of lashes. Her ballooned lips are so beesting swollen, they're in another time zone. I know it's evil of me but I have to take a quick photo. She doesn't notice, but security does. They grab me and dump me out on the street. My kids tell me I've totally embarrassed them, but I think they secretly like it when I embarrass them. When I break rules, I'm myself again. This is when they see mommy has returned.

16 June 2022

Therapy class

There's a therapy group called Self Compassion. At first I used to heckle the teacher. I wondered, how can they teach self compassion to us, when we're crueller to ourselves than anyone else? We're the first to slap that stigma label on us. Today I feel different about the therapist. With the help of the shrink, I've come to the conclusion that this illness is not my fault. I didn't choose my parents or my circumstances. For that alone I'm giving myself some compassion, so rather than heckling, I'm now taking notes in the compassion therapy class. I can't believe I'm writing this down.

1 When shame comes up in your mind, slap the label 'shame' on it. This distances you from the pain and stops the endless

stories you make up about why you're ashamed, and whose fault it is you've got it.

2 When you feel shame, investigate where you sense it in your body. What kind of sensations are they? Replace judgement with curiosity. When you focus on the sensations you can become more like a scientist studying what's in a petri dish, less like a victim.

3 Sometimes unconsciously, people recreate familiar situations that keep the shame going. It's the devil they know. Speak to yourself like you would a friend. Ask yourself what actions you could suggest taking to avoid falling into the trap of feeling even more shame.

There is another therapy group called Emotional Regulation Management. We had to write down what we feel in our bodies when someone hits one of our triggers. The idea is that if we can identify those feelings as they're 'coming down the pipeline', we can choose better ways to express them. These are my top three triggers:

1 Rage feels like a thunderstorm of lightning bolts thrashing it out in my chest. I wonder how many innocent people I've blamed for those bolts.

2 Envy feels like there's a dull, aching heating pad over my heart and something thorny caught in my throat. As soon as I feel those, I'm on the prowl for someone that has what I want.

3 Isolation and abandonment is a twanging of my heart strings. It starts the old theme tune playing, 'I'm a freak and if people found out who I really am, they'd run.'

After I identified those emotions, the therapist told me to thank them because they meant well. They were part of my survival kit. So I thanked them. My anger because it got me away from my parents; my envy because it motivated me to become successful; and my isolation because it pushed me to always find a community.

I feel a little like I'm swallowing the kool-aid but it makes me feel better, so I'm drinking it.

We have a library here which I've passed about six times a day and never noticed. For me not to look in every door to see what's going on is a sure sign I haven't been well. So today – big progress! – I looked around the door. There seemed to be lots of books on the shelves. I couldn't think why until the word 'library' floated into my head. I went in, took a book from the shelves, opened it up and found I could actually read words. Before this, I didn't know what all those letters, jumping around on the page, were supposed to mean.

Of all the books I could have chosen that day, I picked the one completely relevant to my situation. It was called *Falling Upward*, by Richard Rohr. These were the words that first caught my attention:

'*We have two tasks in our lives. In the first half we establish an identity, a home, relationships, friends, community and security. This first-half-of-life task is no more than finding the starting gate. We all need some successes and positive feedback early in life, or will spend the rest of our lives demanding it or bemoaning its lack from others. There is a good and needed narcissism. You first have to have an ego structure to then let go of it and move beyond it.*'

I took the book back to my room, and kept reading. '*You*

cannot walk the second half of life's journey with first journey tools. You need a whole new tool kit.'

Rohr wrote that the second half of life is where you can get a wider perspective of life. He calls that a 'larger container', and says we experience this larger container as our identification moves from 'I' and expands into 'we' or 'us'. This larger container can hold anxiety, stress, rage, pain, boredom – whatever is incoming – without us having to react to them. Rohr said we're capable of so much more than our previously narrow view of who we are; that our container is so much wider than this identity as an 'I'.

Having a wider container means you're able to stand back and observe your thoughts and feelings instead of just being dragged into their drama. If you observe anger it's different from *being* angry. You can say, 'There is anger' rather than, 'I'm angry'. Finally, an instruction manual on how to live my life.

When I'm in that 'open space' frame of mind, I feel like I'm in Montana again underneath that open Big Sky. I also felt it in Spirit Rock: everything inside me suddenly went still, and a feeling of warmth began to spread through my heart and stomach. Thoughts and emotions entered and exited without me interfering. It's like observing your breath going in and out; it doesn't need you to think about it, it just breathes automatically.

I just allowed life to carry me along without a struggle. If that's not flowing, nothing is.

Rohr says with practice we can leave the first half of life, which is all about building an ego, and go on to the second half, which is about tearing it down. With the release of the ego, there's space to be able to hold other people's feelings.

If you're too self-involved, you can't feel empathy for someone. When people feel that state of openness, they often experience a new sense of belonging or coming home.

'If you can hold it all inside this bigger container, you'll give the pain space and it will lose its contraction and often the pain decreases.'

In my first half, I had ambition. I was served with hot and cold running success. When I was younger, I lived with my foot on the accelerator to chase what I wanted and assumed I'd get it if I pushed hard enough. This is why you have to be young to be able to tolerate all those high speeds and late nights. Maybe it's good I'm older now. (I can't believe I just said that.)

So many of us (me) try to keep the first half our permanent home, mostly to keep out the fear of – dare I use the word? – death? With a bigger container, you're free from those upsetting concepts by inviting thoughts and feelings in even if they're unpleasant by saying, 'Come on in boys and girls, there's room at the inn.'

If you hold on to the first half of your life, you'll only get more and more discontent because it's a losing game. If looks were your thing, people stop looking. If success was your thing, you'll always be replaced by someone younger. That's not just television. That's the law of the jungle.

18 June 2022

I was supposed to leave the clinic today but begged to stay one more day. Ed is going to have to drag me out by my ankles, I feel so happy here, but I know I'm going to have to face outside sooner or later.

19 June 2022

Ed picks me up and he has to do about forty trips up and down the stairs to get all the suitcases out of the building. He needs to pack up all the items I requested over the month which I never wore or ate. It was like I was moving house. I almost broke down when Risk and I hugged goodbye but we both said we hoped we'd never see each other again.

*

In the next few days, to celebrate my return to life, I went bicycling through Italy with two girlfriends, Mary-Lu and Amanda. We'd arranged it before I was in the clinic. They had assumed I wouldn't be going on the trip after all, but I felt so good after leaving the clinic that I asked to join them. We rode thirty miles a day from Naples down the coast of Italy. I wasn't looking for anything in particular; not meaning, not peace, not an epiphany, and by letting all that go, for the next five days I felt completely free. My face smiled for the first time in months. I felt like a stream was rushing through every part of me. I took my feet off the pedals and let gravity pull me down the sides of mountains. As the wind rushed past my face, I could smell pine trees, heat, herbs and flowers. And if that's not 'flowing', I don't know what is.

We went to tiny villages nestled in the crevices of mountains. The town squares were full of locals. They had such a great appetite for life, so free, like they were eating life. In the crowded cafés, babies were crawling through everyone's legs; on the balconies, old people were hanging their sheets to dry, while their neighbours were leaning over them to gossip. In one village we went to, a brass band was playing in the town square as statues of Jesus were being carried through the cobbled streets by bent-over priests.

I thought you could never be lonely in one of these tightly bound communities: everyone mingled and no one was left out. I told Ed we should move there permanently and join the old people drying their sheets. Ed said 'No', again.

I visited other places on my bucket list. I wasn't looking for meaning; I just wanted to go to visit people and places that make me feel good. I went to Woodstock, New York – a left-over from the 60s – to stay with Neil Gaiman, a friend from way back when he was nothing. ('BC', before he was a cult.) On day one, I asked him where to find the occult shops. He said every shop in Woodstock is an occult shop, and true enough every shop was filled to the hilt with every witch accessory you could dream of. You need an eye of newt? A pinkie fingernail from a virgin? Recipes for revenge? They got it – on sale. Tinctures up the wazoo.

I went to use the loo in the County Hall where there was a dance class of older folks doing the Charleston. They beckoned me to join, which I did, and after the class we went to some-one's house for a party, with cake and water-pistol fights. Neil called, as I was missing in action for the day, but I told him I was on a roll and had no time for him. This again is the America I love, 'where the deer and the buffalo and eccentrics play'. From there I kept on driving, this time to the virgin backwoods of Maine. Maine has not been Starbucked to death . . . yet. Most of America is lined with McDonald's, Pizza Hut, Burger King and nail bars every few feet until you hit Maine. Then suddenly it's all forest and lakes and sparsely dotted log cabins or white shingled Victorian homes with an American flag plonked in the front yard.

I went to Maine with my close friend Rahla Xenopoulos, and we stayed in a treehouse. It had sunlight gold shafts streaking through the branches, and a path leading to a sparkling navy blue river. The other homes hidden in the trees belonged either to the luckiest people in the world or wood elves. I took a kayak out to the middle of the river. The silence was so complete, you could hear a fish jump miles away. I was just sitting there bobbing slightly on the ripples, when suddenly, from out of the trees, a bald American eagle took off like a 747, and my jaw hit the floor of the kayak. He looked just as majestic and pissed off as he does on the American dollar bill with his sharp hooked nose and slit eyes. Appearing very arrogant, rich and . . . American. It suddenly took off and my heart skipped beats. Those wings, flapping away in slow-mo, probably spanned about seven feet. As I paddled off in pure bliss, don't think it didn't occur to me to kayak into the sun and disappear forever. I was in the 'flowing' but apparently not in the 'knowing', because two miles later I was lost.

I went on these trips to Italy, Woodstock, Maine, not to find meaning this time but just to feel happy. I was like someone who just got their sight back after being blind.

As far as finding a home, I'm not going to end up in some homey nest in the country pottering around – God, I hate that word – in the garden, making jam and having lovely teas and scones with masses of yummy cream with my scrummy neighbours. It ain't happening.

If I can build a bigger container, that'll be my home, and the good news is it's portable and it goes wherever I go. And physically if I end up on a dude ranch in Colorado, an eco house in Findhorn or a witch's coven in Woodstock – all things are possible. Ed may even like moving to one of those. Who knows?

Remember I said earlier I wanted to meet a wise woman? At this point, I'm thinking, I'm the right age and if I stopped dyeing my hair, I could qualify.

Afterword

At first I thought writing a book about meaning was something you'd do when you reached the last act of your life and were close to shuffling off your mortal coil. But I changed my mind. I think people of all ages began asking themselves after the Covid lockdown, 'How do I want to live my life?' Some of the people I've met on my travels, much younger people, told me they're yearning for a more profound life, that they don't want the usual get married/make money/have kids/become boring life. They want something less conventional, like maybe living closer to nature and showing it some respect. The old beliefs that success, fame and money bring us peace and happiness have crumbled like the Berlin Wall. And, as it turns out, meaning might be the only thing worth looking for.

Last week I went back to Findhorn, the place in Scotland I wrote about in my last book. It's an eco-village with a population of about 600. It's 'eco' because the people there are trying to be environmentally less harmful than the rest of the human race and they've been trying for the last sixty years. There's car sharing, large whirly wind turbines, big-time biomass, solar-panelled homes – some with lawns growing on the roofs to keep the heat in – and huge vegetable gardens where I sometimes worked in the mornings. This is a woman (me) who does not touch plants or dirt, who could wave at them but never touch them. But a new side of my personality had been uncorked. Here, I'm known as the 'tomato demon'.

Because of my OCD, I can pick dozens of tomatoes in seconds. I enjoy working near my fellow gardeners: they're earthy but with a sense of humour which they need to tolerate me. You know by now how much I love blending in and being accepted? When someone told me to go pick weeds, I was thrilled to get the assignment, and thought I was becoming an asset. I came back with a wheelbarrow full of what I thought were weeds, only to be informed I had dug up all the rocket lettuce which (excuse me) looked exactly the same.

My residence was Rainbow Lodge in the Field of Dreams (how's that for an address?). I lived above a healing centre again, the same one as when I did the Louis Theroux interview. I could just walk down the stairs and pick a healer, any healer. I was at the very tip of the A-frame building, and there was a triangular wall of glass through which I could look into other people's windows at night.

Watching people who don't know they're being observed is far better than any theatre. It's human life being improvised.

The sunsets in Findhorn are almost blinding; a ball of orange flame like the sky is on fire. In the distance I'm able to see the ocean, and nearby there are fields of evergreens swaying from the wind as if they're doing the Hula. Nature is everywhere. On any given hour I can look at cloud formations changing mood moment-to-moment: sometimes wispy grey, then black when they're about to let it rip storm-wise. Those are closely followed by big fluffy cotton candy clouds against a backdrop of bright baby blue sky.

As we bicycle through the village down higgledy-piggledy walkways, cocooned by flowers and trees, everyone I pass smiles at me. Not that 'have a nice day' fake one, but from deep down they're zapping happiness at you; so you zap it back. I could see the ocean.

I ride my bike next to the water, with sailboats bobbing and stone pubs and still everyone smiles because they live in this mecca – what's to not smile about? No souvenir stands in sight or any sign of selling out.

The shrink is wearing the perfect clothes today. But don't forget, I only see her top half so I'm judging her from the waist up. She's in a grey woollen turtleneck and it makes her look very chic. My mother would approve.

I'm doing most of the talking today because I won't see her again until after I've handed in this book. I have three more days to my deadline. I've been up for many, many days.

R: *I was thinking how to end this book because I have to stick to the truth of what's happened. I'm not a fiction writer. I can't fake it. I mean I could say I rode into the sunset but it would be a lie, and life isn't like that unless you're a cowboy.*

I have to tell you, reading Rohr's book was the most profound thing that happened to me, besides you.

(I added this quickly; I don't want the shrink to not like me.)

Developing this larger container has given me hope. Best of all is learning that I'm much more than my emotions. I'm not my anger.

S: *Sometimes you need some anger otherwise you'll be taken advantage of. There's the other extreme. Sometimes people get in the habit of going limp when they're threatened. That isn't a helpful response either.*

R: *Yeah, that's true, limping isn't going to help when you're getting mugged. That's when you need to give it some welly. What exactly does welly mean? I just said it without knowing.*

S: *It comes from the Scottish Highland Games. They hold a contest to see who can throw a welly the furthest. The person who wins is the one who puts the most energy into the toss. Any more than that, I don't know. Maybe you should look it up.*

R: *I'm not going to look it up, I like that explanation. Maybe I should start a contest to see who can throw their socks the furthest? So people can, 'Give it some sock.'*

(She laughed. I can't believe it.)

S: *I think that's where something like Acceptance and Commitment Therapy was interesting. They say even if you're seventy years old, you have to learn to accept things as they are, because no matter how much you resist, you can't change it. So you think, 'Okay, what kind of seventy-year-old do I want to be?' Not accepting it is the root to psychological distress. And the second thing is learning to be flexible. Not saying to yourself, 'Well, that didn't work so I'm a complete failure.' You have to learn to tolerate when you're being let down. When they were working on the Hadron Collider in Switzerland, and it wasn't successful, those scientists had beaming smiles on their faces. They were excited because they were learning what doesn't work. They tried something and it failed so they can now cross that off their list. They don't think, 'We tried that experiment and it didn't work so we're all failures.' If we could just think like that, 'I'll try it and if it doesn't work, I can try something else.'*

R: *I'll tell you one thing that's changed in me. I don't feel any fear any more about what's coming. Even though I may change in the next ten minutes and life may become more painful again, I'm not scared like I was. This idea of having a second half makes me so jazzed up to reinvent again but for something much deeper than before. I thought it was all over at this point in my life, but this second half seems way more interesting than the first.*

S: *I've noticed a big change in you. It's been exciting to observe you moving from desperation to where you are now. Having seen you in that place when you were in such despair, saying, 'I'm useless and have no point. I feel like killing myself.' And you've been able to move from that place to this place now. I'd say, right now you're well into the second half of your life.*

R: *Well, you've done a good job.*

S: *You've done a good job, too. I created a frame within which you either could or could not have done the work. And you did it. It's not over, of course. Getting to know yourself with kindness, viewing yourself with compassion, is an ongoing process. You were so harsh on yourself at the beginning; almost all the time. What are you going to do after you hand in the book?*

R: *I just want to have a good time for a while. I've always felt guilty about doing that, always pushing myself too hard mostly to prove a point to my dad. I just want a little joy. Is that asking too much?*

S: *Watch it, because the chase for happiness can also lead to desperation.*

R: *I don't care. I was in a mental institution for six weeks. This is my version of popping the champagne and blowing up the balloons. It's my farewell party to the first half of my life and welcoming me into the second.*

Index

INDEX

AND NOW FOR THE GOOD NEWS . . . :
THE MUCH-NEEDED TONIC FOR OUR FRAZZLED WORLD
RUBY WAX

As we begin to see the green shoots of a post-pandemic world, Ruby Wax's clever and witty *And Now for the Good News* is the blueprint we all need for achieving a kinder, more compassionate world.

Brimming with practical learnings, Ruby gives readers the opportunity to create lasting positive change and provides us all with a much-needed tonic for better mental health.

She spent three years speaking to the people who are spearheading the latest innovation and influencing a brighter future for humanity. From the communities being designed to eradicate loneliness and the companies putting their employees' happiness first, to the impressive AI technology teaching children with learning difficulties and taking literacy levels higher than ever before. *And Now for the Good News* distils her inspiring findings into key practical takeaways for all.

Ruby's here to equip us all with a positive roadmap for a brighter world and, most importantly, for better mental well-being.

'This book couldn't be more needed right now!'

Nigella Lawson

'Ruby has a uniquely vibrant and clever way of thinking'

Elizabeth Day

HOW TO BE HUMAN: THE MANUAL
RUBY WAX

It took us 4 billion years to evolve to where we are now. No question, anyone reading this has won the evolutionary Hunger Games by the fact you're on all twos and not some fossil. This should make us all the happiest species alive – most of us aren't, what's gone wrong? We've started treating ourselves more like machines and less like humans. We're so used to upgrading things like our iPhones: as soon as the new one comes out, we don't think twice, we dump it. (Many people I know are now on iWife4 or iHusband8, the motto being if it's new, it's better.)

We can't stop the future from arriving, no matter what drugs we're on. But even if nearly every part of us becomes robotic, we'll still, fingers crossed, have our minds, which, hopefully, we'll be able use for things like compassion, rather than chasing what's 'better', and if we can do that we're on the yellow brick road to happiness.

I wrote this book with a little help from a monk, who explains how the mind works, and also gives some mindfulness exercises, and a neuroscientist who explains what makes us 'us' in the brain. We answer every question you've ever had about: evolution, thoughts, emotions, the body, addictions, relationships, kids, the future and compassion.

How to be Human is extremely funny, true and the only manual you'll need to help you upgrade your mind as much as you've upgraded your iPhone.

'With this marvellous book, Ruby Wax has confirmed her position as one of the most readable, inspirational and engaging writers in the field of human mental health, happiness and fulfilment'

Stephen Fry

'*How to be Human* is, without exaggeration, a lifeline; wise, pratical and funny, it is a handbook for those in despair. It is actually for everyone alive, for the curious, or disillusioned or muddled or just plain happy'

Joanna Lumley

A MINDFULNESS GUIDE FOR THE FRAZZLED
RUBY WAX

'We are frazzled, all of us . . .'

Five hundred years ago no one died of stress: we invented this concept and now we let it rule us.

In *A Mindfulness Guide for the Frazzled*, Ruby Wax shows us how to de-frazzle for good by making simple changes that give us time to breathe, reflect and live in the moment. It's an easy-to-understand introduction to mindfulness, weaved together with Ruby's trademark wit and humour.

Let Ruby be your guide to a healthier, happier you. You've nothing to lose but your stress . . .

'Ruby Wax has written a guide to mindfulness that's as hilarious as it is useful'

Arianna Huffington

'Whip-smart on the subject . . . she teaches the art of doing nothing in a way that doesn't send you to sleep'

The Times

'A wonderful book full of passion, verve and humour'

Mark Williams, author of
*Mindfulness: A Practical
Guide to Finding Peace in a
Frantic World*